全国中医药行业高等教育"十四五"创新教材

医学综合英语

（供中医学、中药学、中西医临床医学等专业用）

主 编 刘 潜 周志刚

全国百佳图书出版单位
中国中医药出版社
·北 京·

图书在版编目（CIP）数据

医学综合英语 / 刘潜，周志刚主编 . — 北京：
中国中医药出版社，2023.12
全国中医药行业高等教育"十四五"创新教材
ISBN 978 – 7 – 5132 – 6077 – 0

Ⅰ . ①医… Ⅱ . ①刘… ②周… Ⅲ . ①医学—英语—
中医学院—教材 Ⅳ . ① R

中国国家版本馆 CIP 数据核字（2023）第 231112 号

中国中医药出版社出版

北京经济技术开发区科创十三街 31 号院二区 8 号楼
邮政编码 100176
传真 010－64405721
廊坊市佳艺印务有限公司印刷
各地新华书店经销

开本 787×1092 1/16 印张 14.75 字数 487 千字
2023 年 12 月第 1 版 2023 年 12 月第 1 次印刷
书号 ISBN 978 – 7 – 5132 – 6077 – 0

定价 69.00 元
网址 www.cptcm.com

服 务 热 线 010－64405510
购 书 热 线 010－89535836
维 权 打 假 010－64405753

微信服务号 zgzyycbs
微商城网址 https://kdt.im/LIdUGr
官 方 微 博 http://e.weibo.com/cptcm
天猫旗舰店网址 https://zgzyycbs.tmall.com

如有印装质量问题请与本社出版部联系（010－64405510）

全国中医药行业高等教育"十四五"创新教材

《医学综合英语》编委会

编写说明

党的十八大以来，中医药参与共建"一带一路"取得积极进展。中医药已传播至 196 个国家和地区，成为中国与东盟、欧盟、非盟、拉共体等组织合作的重要领域。第七十二届世界卫生大会审议通过了《国际疾病分类第十一次修订本（ICD—11）》，首次纳入以中医药为主体的传统医学章节，中医药历史性地进入世界主流医学体系，中医药在国际传统医学领域的话语权和影响力显著提升。

党和政府重视中医药的海外发展。中共中央国务院印发的《关于促进中医药传承创新发展的意见》再次强调，要推动中医药文化海外传播。国家中医药管理局印发的《中医药高质量共建"一带一路"发展规划（2021—2025年）》提出"深化国际组织框架下合作"，"深化与其他国际组织、其他传统医学机构交流与合作"。2017 年 10 月，习近平总书记在十九大报告中提出"坚持中西医并重，传承发展中医药事业"，2019 年 10 月《关于促进中医药传承创新发展的意见》又提出"坚持中西医并重，推动中医药和西医药相互补充、协调发展"，这需要中医与西医相互学习、相互借鉴。

中医药院校的学生不仅肩负着传承与创新中医药的使命，同时也承担着未来对外交流先进医学成果及传播中医药文化的责任。医学英语（English for Medical Purpose，EMP）作为专门用途英语（English for Specific Purposes，ESP）的分枝之一，在中医药文化海外传播方面和与医学同行的交流、学习中不可或缺。对于高等医学院校的学生来说，了解国际医学的前沿动向，进行国际学术交流，以便更好地撰写高质量学术论文，或与国外专家无障碍地进行科学研究、临床实践的学术交流，或到国外高校访问、学习、深造，这些都离不开医学英语。

基于以上背景，《医学综合英语》立足于临床，纲目并举，以各科临床为纲，以听、说、写、读、词汇为目。本教材分为 10 章，覆盖临床各科，每章以听、说、写、读为章节框架，提升学生医学英语的实际应用能力。在听、说部分，本教材根据"目标情景"需要，我们按章节内容需要设计一个个临床故事，把临床实践中常用的句型及术语充分展现出来，让学生在听故事中学习。在阅读理解部分，我们根据"学习需求"，采用来自英美国家临床病历的素材再现临床情景，语言比较地道。另外，考虑到医学的特殊性，本书将医学术语的词根、词根含义、词例及词例概念以表格形式列举出来，方便学生查阅及记忆。为充分体现医学术语的趣味性，我们也设计了短小而简单的临床故事，让学生在临床故事中学习医学英语术语。在口语部分，我们以角色扮演的形式让学生自由发挥以展现所学知识。除此之外，我们还每章提供一个临床病例，要求学生讨论后回答，以锻炼学生的临床分析能力和思维能力。在写作部分，我们以临床病历写作为手段，将病历写作分解成 10 个部分，在每个部分详述写作要点，并举例说明。为方便学生在学习过程中查阅临床各科术语，我们在每章末尾提供了各科的疾病名称及相关系统的术语。

本教材编写工作的具体分工如下：第一章由周志刚、巢波、洪子杰编写，第二章由刘潜、周平生编写，第三章由蔡少华、戴颖恒、张敏编写，第四章由徐华、陈琪、张榕编写，第五章由张海萍、周凌云、陈静茹编写，第六章由皮冬平、成国春、胡天翔编写，第七章由吴江、黄丽娟、顾楠等编写，第八章由彭爱芬、周紫煜、涂雅雯等编写，第九章由周志刚、王梦霞、梅琳等编写，第十章由黄之静、辜茜等编写。

因本教材编写团队水平有限，若有不当之处，敬请批评指正。

《医学综合英语》编委会
2023 年 12 月

Catalog

Chapter 1

General Introduction

Section A   Focus Listening

Conversation

Listen to the dialogue and fill in the blanks with proper words.

M=mother, D=doctor

(A young mother rushed into the emergency room, holding a kid in her arms)

M: Help, Doctor. My son almost can't breathe, hurry up please!

D: Take it easy! Madam, tell me what happened to your kid?

M: You see, my son has been in paroxysmal _____ with wheezing, difficulty in breathing, cough and chest tightness.

D: When did it begin?

M: About 2 hours ago, he told me he felt uncomfortable. Soon after, he opened his mouth to breathe laboriously, and got worse later. That's why I hurried to come here.

D: Does he cough seriously? Much _____? Or running a temperature?

M: Yes, he coughed up a lot of sputum, white and foamy. But he didn't run a temperature.

D: Did you notice a cyanosis on his lips?

M: Cyanosis? But I found his lips were blue and purple.

D: That is cyanosis.

M: Oh.

D: OK. Let him sit upright, I'd like to examine his lung and heart.

M: Doctor, can you do something for my boy first?

D: Don't worry, I need several minutes to examine him before taking any measures.

M: OK, I see.

The doctor examined the lady's son.

D: There are extensive wheezing sounds in both lungs and trachea, prolonged _____ and the heart rate is 108 beats/min，I'm sure your son suffer from asthma, his symptoms will be relieved immediately after he is treated with nebulized salbutamol.

A few minutes later, the lady's son can breathe smoothly.

M: Thank you very much!

D: That's all right, but I need to know his history.

M: No problem!

D: Have these similar symptoms happened before?

M: No, never happened before. It's the first time, I was frightened!

D: Does anything special _____. For example, cold, special food, or pollen?

M: I have no idea, but my mother took him to Bayi Park this afternoon, you know lots of pigeons are there, it's spectacular! He has an episode of paroxysmal dyspnea now. Does it relate to the pigeons?

D: Possibly, you know the animal hair or mites are also asthma allergens. Please go to the pulmonary function examination room and clinical laboratory with these two test sheets. I'll assess the condition based on the test results.

About half an hour later, the mother and her son came back with test results.

M: Doctor, here are the results, is it serious?

D: Let me see, the examination reveals: FEV1 is diminished to 72% of the normal and diminished PEF, the arterial blood gas analysis reads: diminished PaO_2, both _____ function examination and arterial blood gas analysis are in accordance with diagnosis of medium asthma.

M: I heard asthma was hard to be cured, will it affect my son's growth?

D: No, it doesn't, but I think you should pay attention to two points: Firstly, exposure to allergen should be averted. Secondly, exacerbation should be prevented from happening, your son should receive persistent treatment as early as possible in case of the acute asthma attack.

New Words & Expressions

wheezing 气喘　　　　　　　　　　cyanosis 发绀
trachea 气管　　　　　　　　　　　nebulize 使……成雾状，使成喷雾状
salbutamol 沙丁胺醇　　　　　　　　allergen 过敏原
FEV1 第 1 秒用力呼气容积　　　　　PEF 最大呼气流量

Passage

Answer the questions after listening to the passage.

1. What is the average body temperature?

A. 105 °F .

B. 98.6 °F .

C. 37.5℃ .

D. Both B and C.

2. What does the term Homeostasis refers to?

A. Constant internal environment.

B. Variable internal environment.

C. Changing external environment.

D. None of them.

3. What are the types of feedback in homeostasis?

A. Negative feedback.

B. Positive feedback.

C. Feed-forward feedback.

D. Both A and B.

4. Heat from the body is lost in the form of_____.

A. sweating.

B. shivering.

C. inhalation.

D. defecation.

5. What happens to the body when there is failure in homeostasis?

A. No change.

B. Development of disease.

C. Disappearance of disease.

D. None of the above.

Section B   Reading Comprehension

Text

A 17-year-old girl was transferred to this hospital because of chest pain and hemoptysis. She had been well except for mild asthma until 4 months earlier, when pedal edema developed, testing revealed (3+) proteinuria, hematuria, and hyperlipidemia. One month later, a renal biopsy was performed at another facility, and a diagnosis of membranous glomerulonephritis was made. Testing for antibodies to hepatitis B and hepatitis C, as well as anti-ribonuclear protein, anti-topoisomerase I, anti-Smith antibody, anti-Ro (SS-A), anti-La (SS-B), anti-double-stranded DNA, and anti-nuclear antibody was negative. The levels of serum C3 and C4 complement were normal. Enalapril, atorvastatin, and fluid restriction began; after the therapy for several weeks, the patient stopped taking atorvastatin because of muscle pain. After the renal biopsy, she had persistent pain in the back and abdomen. Ultrasonography of the kidney disclosed a small perinephric hematoma.

Over the course of the next 2 months, although imaging studies showed diminution in the size of the hematoma, the patient continued to report severe pain in the back as well as abdominal pain, which lasted despite treatment with oxycodone and acetaminophen and interfered with her activities and sleep, and thus she largely stayed in bed. Bilateral lower leg edema occurred intermittently. During the 2 weeks before admission, pain in the back and abdomen decreased in intensity, but she began to have pain in the chest, radiating to the neck and shoulder, which was exacerbated by coughing and deep inspiration.

Six days before admission, she was seen in a pain clinic at another hospital; a diagnosis of neuralgia of the intercostal nerves was made, and gabapentin and tramadol were prescribed. Over the next several days the pain worsened, cough and hemoptysis developed, and one episode of dyspnea occurred, which was relieved with the use of an albuterol (salbutamol) inhaler.

The day before admission, she went to a second hospital because of increasing chest pain. The temperature was 39.0℃, the blood pressure 115/69 mmHg, the pulse 156 beats per minute (bpm), and the respiratory rate 50 breaths per minute. Oxygen saturation was 98% while the patient was breathing ambient air. On examination, her breathing was shallow because of chest pain. The lungs were clear, and the results of the physical examination were otherwise normal. Two liters of normal saline were administered in the emergency room, and the patient was admitted to the pediatric intensive care unit. Treatment with enoxaparin was begun. The oxygen saturation intermittently fell to 92%~93% and oxygen was administered by nasal cannula at 1~2 liters per minute. Urinalysis results were positive for protein (3+) and for blood (2+), and revealed a specific gravity of 1.041. Chest radiography revealed a patchy density in the left costophrenic angle and electrocardiography showed sinus tachycardia. Morphine sulfate was administered for the patient's pain, and specimens of blood were sent for culture.

The next day, transthoracic echocardiography showed moderate right ventricular dilatation with an estimated pulmonary artery pressure of 60 mm Hg; flattened, paradoxical septal motion; and a small pericardial effusion. No intraatrial or intraventricular clot was identified. After prophylactic treatment with acetylcysteine and bicarbonate, spiral computed tomographic (CT) scanning and CT angiography of the chest were performed. There were emboli in both pulmonary arteries with multiple bilateral pulmonary infarcts and small bilateral pleural effusions. Renal ultrasonography revealed a hematoma around the left kidney; Doppler studies showed no clot in the inferior vena cava, and noninvasive testing of the legs did not reveal deep venous thromboses. Enoxaparin was discontinued, and treatment with heparin was begun; the patient was transferred to this hospital and admitted to the intensive care unit.

She had mild intermittent asthma, which required occasional use of an albuterol inhaler, with upper respiratory infections, but was otherwise well and had not been hospitalized previously. She was a good student in high school and did not use tobacco, alcohol, or illicit drugs. Her mother had multiple sclerosis and asthma, her father had hypertension, and distant cousins had systemic lupus erythematosus. A paternal cousin was receiving dialysis for an unknown cause, her mother and two siblings carried the sickle cell trait, and her fraternal twin was in good health. The patient had taken oral contraceptives for the past 3 years, for treatment of irregular menses. On transfer, her medications included heparin, morphine, ranitidine, albuterol, and dextrose normal saline.

On admission, the temperature was 38.3℃, the pulse 148 beats per minute, the blood pressure 138/72 mmHg, the respiratory rate 34 breaths per minute, and the oxygen saturation 92% while the patient was breathing ambient air. There was decreased inspiratory effort and a prominent second heart sound. Jugular venous pulsations, measured with the patient in a reclining position at 30 degrees, were 7 cm above the sternal angle. A pulmonary artery tap, a right ventricular heave, and a harsh systolic murmur (grade 2/6) over the left lower sternal border were heard. There was tenderness in the right mid-abdomen and 1+ edema of both legs extending up to the knees.

Electrocardiography revealed an S wave in lead I and Q and T waves in lead Ⅲ. A management decision was made.

New Words & Expressions

hemoptysis [hɪˈmɒptəsɪs] *n.* expectoration of blood from some part of the respiratory tract 咳血

pedal [ˈped(ə)l] *a.* of or relating to the feet 足的，脚的

proteinuria [prəʊtiˈnjʊərɪə] *n.* the presence of excess protein in the urine 蛋白尿

hematuria [ˌhiməˈtjurɪə] *n.* the presence of blood or blood cells in the urine 血尿

hyperlipidemia [ˌhaɪpərlɪˈpidi:mɪə] *n.* the presence of excess fat or lipids in the blood 高脂血症

glomerulonephritis [gləʊmerjʊləʊnefˈraɪtɪs] *n.* nephritis marked by inflammation of the capillaries of the renal glomeruli 肾小球肾炎

enalapril [eˈnælæprɪl] *n.* an antihypertensive drug $C_{20}H_{28}N_2O_5$ that is an ACE inhibitor administered orally in the form of its maleate 依那普利

atorvastatin [ətɔ:rˈvɑ:steɪtɪn] *n.* 阿托伐他汀（降血脂药）

ultrasonography [ʌltrəsəˈnɒgrəfɪ] *n.* a test in which high-frequency sound waves (ultrasound) are bounced off tissues and the echoes are converted into a picture (sonogram) 超声波检查

hematoma [ˌhiːməˈtəʊmə] *n.* a mass of usually clotted blood that forms in a tissue, organ, or body space as a result of a broken blood vessel 血肿

oxycodone [ˌɒksɪˈkəʊdəʊn] *n.* 羟考酮（药）

acetaminophen [əˌsiːtəˈmɪnəfən] *n.* 对乙酰氨基酚

intercostal [ɪntəˈkɒstl] *n.* situated or extending between the ribs 肋间的

tramadol [ˈtræmædɔl] *n.* a synthetic opioid analgesic administered orally in the form of its hydrochloride $C_{16}H_{25}NO_2 \cdot HCl$ to treat moderate to severe pain 曲马多

gabapentin [ˌgæbəˈpentin] *n.* a new kind of anti-convulsion medicine with good tolerance 加巴喷丁

enoxaparin [eˈnɒksəpərɪn] *n.* 依诺肝素

cannula [ˈkænjʊlə] *n.* a small tube for insertion into a body cavity or into a duct or vessel 插管，套管

transthoracic [ˌtrænsθəˈræsɪk] *n.* done or made by way of the thoracic cavity 经胸廓的

tomography [təˈmɒgrəfi] *n.* X 线体层照相机；X 线断层照相装置

acetylcysteine [æsɪtɪlˈsɪstiːɪn] *n.* 乙酰半胱氨酸

lupus [ˈlupəs] *n.* one of several diseases that affect the skin and joints 狼疮

erythematous [ˌerɪˈθiːmətəs] *n.* a disorder characterized by skin inflammation 红斑狼疮

inspiratory [ɪnˈspaɪrətərɪ] *a.* of, relating to, used for, or associated with inspiration 吸入的，吸气的

sternal [ˈstɜːnəl] *a.* of or relating to the sternum 胸骨的；近胸骨的

Exercise

Decide whether the following statements are true (T) or false (F) according to the passage.

_____1. The girl, transferred to this hospital because of chest pain and hemoptysis, had been well except for glomerulonephritis until 14 months earlier.

_____2. Before admission, the patient had pain in the low back and abdomen which was decreased in intensity, then the patient began to have chest pains.

_____3. One episode of dyspnea occurred to the patient, which was relieved with the use of an albuterol inhaler.

_____4. There were no emboli in both pulmonary arteries with multiple bilateral pulmonary infarcts and small bilateral pleural effusions before admission.

_____5. The patient's mother and two siblings carried the sickle cell trait, and her fraternal twin was in good health.

Answer the following questions according to the passage.

1. What medicine was prescribed when a diagnosis of neuralgia of the intercostal nerves was made six days before admission?

_____

2. How many hospitals did the patient go before she was admitted in the intensive care unit?

_____

3. What were the patient's vital signs on admission?

_____

Use the appropriate form of the words or phrases in the box to complete the following sentences.

contraceptives	dialysis	oxycodone	cavity ultrasonography
thromboses	intermittent	specimens	glomerulonephritis
dilatation	hematuria	pediatric	gabapentin and tramadol

1. If you have _____, a urine test will show up blood and protein in the urine.

2. Serious potential consequences of over-dosage with _____ are central nervous system depression, respiratory depression and death.

3. The patient continued to report severe pain in the back as well as abdominal pain, which lasted despite treatment with _____ and acetaminophen and interfered with her activities and sleep.

4. Two liters of normal saline were administered in the emergency room, and the patient was admitted to the _____ intensive care unit.

5. Morphine sulfate was administered for the patient's pain, and _____ of blood were sent for culture.

6. The next day, transthoracic echocardiography showed moderate right ventricular _____ with an estimated pulmonary artery pressure of 60 mmHg.

7. Doppler studies showed no clot in the inferior vena cava, and noninvasive testing of the legs did not reveal deep venous _____.

8. She had mild _____ asthma, which required occasional use of an albuterol inhaler, with upper respiratory infections.

9. A paternal cousin was receiving _____ for an unknown cause, her mother and two siblings carried the sickle cell trait.

10. The patient has taken oral _____ for treatment of irregular menses for the past 3 years.

Translation

A. Translate the following expressions into English.

1. 肾活检
2. 背部和腹部持续疼痛
3. 氧气饱和度
4. 肺动脉压
5. 下腔静脉
6. 上呼吸道感染
7. 双腿水肿
8. 向上延伸至膝盖

B. Translate the following sentences or expressions into Chinese.

1. Enoxaparin was discontinued, and treatment with heparin was begun; the patient was transferred to this hospital and admitted to the intensive care unit.

2. A pulmonary artery tap, a right ventricular heave, and a harsh systolic murmur (grade 2/6) over the left lower sternal border were heard.

3. After prophylactic treatment with acetylcysteine and bicarbonate, spiral computed tomographic (CT) scanning and CT angiography of the chest were performed.

4. Chest radiography revealed a patchy density in the left costophrenic angle and electrocardiography showed sinus tachycardia.

5. The patient began to have pain in the chest, radiating to the neck and shoulder, which was exacerbated by coughing and deep inspiration.

Section C   Vocabulary (Terminology)

Brief introduction

医学英语词汇是医学专用英语词汇，它是构成英语医学用语的主要部分。如下面的一些英语单词，都属于英语医学词汇的范围。

pneumonia	肺炎
streptococcus	链球菌
arthritis	关节炎
mitral valve	二尖瓣
hemobilia	胆道出血
ejection murmur	喷射性杂音

医学英语的词汇学以医学语言学理论为指导，从词源学、形态学、词义学、词典学角度，系统地介绍医学英语词汇知识，深入分析医学英语词汇的现状及其历史演变过程，并对其发展趋势以及所包含的医学文化知识做出详尽的解释。

医学英语词汇学是英语词汇学的一个分支，其研究对象是医学英语词汇的结构成分、结构规律、结构方式、汉译技巧、表达医学领域中新概念与新事物的新词的创造、医学英语的起源与流变等一系列的相关内容。虽然这些内容与普通词汇、其他科技词汇有不少的共性，但本身仍不失为一个独立的体系。

　　高等医药院校的学生学习医学英语词汇学的目的是通过有关的知识学习，掌握大量的医学词汇，学好医学英语，提高英语水平，参与和促进国际医学交流，发扬祖国的医药事业，为解除患者的痛苦、保障人民身体健康做出更大的贡献。

　　这里我们主要学习医学英语术语。学习医学英语术语的目的也很简单，它包括三个方面的内容：

　　1. 通过将单词分解成不同组成成分来分析　我们学习医学英语时，不要简单地背单词，而是要借助单词分析工具，把一个复杂的单词分解成不同组成部分，如此我们就更容易理解复杂的医学术语。医学英语术语就像玩拼图游戏一样简单，因为医学英语术语是由不同的组成部分组成的具有独一无二的意思的单词。只要你掌握了不同词的组成部分，理解了它的意思，我们就很容易认识这些单词。如：hepatosplenomegaly。

　　hepato- 是 "肝的"；

　　spleno- 是 "脾的"；

　　mega- 是 "巨大的"。

　　所以，hepatosplenomegaly 是 "肝脾肿大的"。

　　2. 把医学术语与人体结构、功能联系起来　术语的记忆应该成为医学生学习的首要任务。本部分的重要内容是如何在健康和疾病的背景下解释这些术语。在合适背景下解释清楚的术语也容易记在脑海里，不容易忘记。例如：hepatitis 是肝的（hepat-）的炎症（-itis），记这个单词只要记两个部分，hepat 是肝，itis 是炎症，把这两个组成部分合在一起就成了肝炎 hepatitis。这样学习单词就可以不需要太多的生物学、解剖学、生理病理学知识。

　　3. 掌握拼写和发音　有些医学术语发音相似，但拼写不同，这主要是由这些术语的意思不同导致的。例如：ilium 和 ileum 发音完全相同，但前者髂骨是骨盆的一部分，而后者是小肠的一部分。有时即使是拼写正确，因为发音错误也可能导致误会。例如：urethra（尿道）是从膀胱至体外的一条管道，但是 ureter（输尿管）是连接肾和膀胱的管道。

Vocabulary (Terminology)

1. 头 head

Combining form	Meaning	Terminology	Terminology meaning
encephalo-	brain	encephalitis	inflammation of the brain 脑炎
cephalo-	head	cephalic	of head 脑的

2. 脸 face

Combining form	Meaning	Terminology	Terminology meaning
facio-	face	facial	on your face or relating to your face 面部的，脸的
prosopo-	face	prosopospasm	面肌痉挛

3. 颊 cheek

Combining form	Meaning	Terminology	Terminology meaning
bucco-	cheek	buccinator	颊肌

4. 颏 chin

Combining form	Meaning	Terminology	Terminology meaning
mento-	chin	mentoplasty	颏成形术

5. 颈 neck, cervix

Combining form	Meaning	Terminology	Terminology meaning
cervico-	neck (of the body or of the uterus)	cervicectomy	a surgical removal of the uterine cervix 子宫切除术

6. 肢 limb, extremity

Combining form	Meaning	Terminology	Terminology meaning
acro-	extremities	acromegaly	enlargement of the extremities 肢端肥大

7. 肩 shoulder

Combining form	Meaning	Terminology	Terminology meaning
omo-	shoulder	omoplate	肩胛骨
scapulo-	scapula (shoulder bone)	scapulalgia	aching of scapula 肩胛痛

8. 肘 elbow

Combining form	Meaning	Terminology	Terminology meaning
cubito-	elbow	cubitoradial	尺桡的

9. 腕 wrist

Combining form	Meaning	Terminology	Terminology meaning
carpo-	wrist bone	carpal tunnel syndrome	腕管综合征

10. 臂 arm

Combining form	Meaning	Terminology	Terminology meaning
brachio-	arm	brachialgia	臂痛

11. 手 hand

Combining form	Meaning	Terminology	Terminology meaning
mano-	hand	manometry	测压法，压力测量法

12. 手指 finger 趾 toe

Combining form	Meaning	Terminology	Terminology meaning
dactylo-	fingers, toes	dactylitis	inflammation of fingers or toes 指、趾炎
digito-	hand, toe	digitoplantar	趾跖的

13. 髋 hip

Combining form	Meaning	Terminology	Terminology meaning
coxo-	hip	coxarthritis	髋关节炎

14. 股 thigh

Combining form	Meaning	Terminology	Terminology meaning
femor/o	femur(thigh bone)	femerocele	Femeral hernia 股疝
mero-	thigh	merocoxalgia	髋股痛

15. 膝 knee

Combining form	Meaning	Terminology	Terminology meaning
genu-	knee	genupetoral position	胸膝位的

16. 踝 ankle

Combining form	Meaning	Terminology	Terminology meaning
malleol/o	ankle	malleotomy	踝切离术，锤骨切开术

17. 足 feet

Combining form	Meaning	Terminology	Terminology meaning
ped/o	foot	podagra	a painful condition of the big toe caused by gout 痛风

18. 足跟 heel, calx

Combining form	Meaning	Terminology	Terminology meaning
calcaneo-	heel bone	calcaneitis	跟骨炎

19. 胸 chest、thorax

Combining form	Meaning	Terminology	Terminology meaning
pecto-	chest	expectorate	to eject from the throat or lungs by coughing or hawking and spitting 咳出
thoraco -	chest	thoracopathy	胸部疾病
stetho-	chest	stethoscope	听诊器

20. 乳房 breast

Combining form	Meaning	Terminology	Terminology meaning
mammo-	breast	mammogram	a photograph of the breasts made by X-rays 乳房 X 线照片
masto-	breast	mastitis	inflammation of the breast or udder usually caused by infection 乳腺炎
mastoido-	mastoid process	mastoiditis	inflammation of the mastoid and especially of the mastoid cells 乳突炎

21. 乳头 nipple, teat

Combining form	Meaning	Terminology	Terminology meaning
papillo-	nipple	papilledema	视神经乳头水肿
thelo	nipple	epithelium	上皮
mammillo-	nipple	mammillitis	乳头炎

22. 膈 diaphragm

Combining form	Meaning	Terminology	Terminology meaning
phreno	diaphragm	phrenospasm	膈痉挛、膈肌痉挛

23. 腹 abdomen, belly

Combining form	Meaning	Terminology	Terminology meaning
abdomin/o	abdomen	abdominocentesis	腹部穿刺
ventro-	belly, side of the body	ventromedial	ventral and medial 腹正中线的
laparo-	abdomen,flank	laparoscopy	visual examination of the abdomen by means of a laparoscope 腹腔镜检查

24. 内脏 viscera, internal organ

Combining form	Meaning	Terminology	Terminology meaning
viscero-	internal organ	viscerosensory	内脏感觉的

25. 腹膜 peritoneum

Combining form	Meaning	Terminology	Terminology meaning
periton(eo)-	peritoneum	peritonitis	腹膜炎

26. 脐 navel, umbilicus

Combining form	Meaning	Terminology	Terminology meaning
omphalo-	umbilicus, navel	omphalorrhagia	脐带出血，脐出血

27. 腹股沟 groin

Combining form	Meaning	Terminology	Terminology meaning
inguino-	groin	inguinodynia	腹股沟痛

28. 腰 loin, waist

Combining form	Meaning	Terminology	Terminology meaning
lumbo-	lower back, lumbus	lumbocostal	腰肋的

29. 骨盆 basin, pelvis

Combining form	Meaning	Terminology	Terminology meaning
pelvi-	pelvis (hipbone)	pelvicellulitis	盆腔蜂窝织炎
pelvo-	hip, pelvic cavity	pelvic	of, relating to, or located in or near the pelvis 骨盆的

30. 背 back

Combining form	Meaning	Terminology	Terminology meaning
dorsi-	back	dorsiflexion	backward(upward) bending of the foot 背屈

31. 尾 tail

Combining form	Meaning	Terminology	Terminology meaning
caudo-	tail	caudalward	向尾端的

Exercise

Please select the proper meaning from column II to match column I.

I	II
(　　) 1. viscer/o	A. lower back
(　　) 2. pelvi-	B. breast
(　　) 3. lumb/o-	C. optic disc(disk); nipple like
(　　) 4. inguin/o-	D. brain
(　　) 5. papillo-	E. internal organ
(　　) 6. ventr/o-	F. pelvis(hipbone)
(　　) 7. encephalo-	G. belly side of the body
(　　) 8. mamm/o	H. groin
(　　) 9. bucco-	I. process on each side of the ankle
(　　) 10. malleol/o	J. cheek
(　　) 11. dactylo-	K. femur(thigh bone)
(　　) 12. cervico-	L. umbilicus, navel

(   ) 13. femor/o   M. fingers, toes

(   ) 14. lapar/o   N. chest

(   ) 15. carpo-   O. neck(of the body or of the uterus)

(   ) 16. omphalo-   P. diaphragm

(   ) 17. pector/o   R. extremities

(   ) 18. phren/o   S. foot

(   ) 19. acro-   T. wrist bone

(   ) 20. ped/o   U. abdomen

Match the following pathological conditions or terms with their meaning below.

periumillical	bronchitis	mastectomy	atrophied	coccygeal
respiratory	strepotcoccemia	pneumococcal	acromegaly	potsis
arthroscopy	inguinal hernia	cystocele	genupetoral	abdominal

1. Sally complained of pain surrounding her umbilicus, the doctor described the pain as _____.

2. The _____ cavity contains digestive organs.

3. Maria's coughing and sneezing was a result of an allergy to animal dander that affected her _____ system.

4. Ms. Daley gave birth to nine children and complained to her doctor about her problems in urinating. After examining, the doctor found her bladder protruding into her vagina due to weakened support system of uterus and bladder and told her she got a _____.

5. Suzy coughed constantly for a week. Her doctor told her that her chest X-ray showed pneumonia. Her sputum (material coughed up from her chest) demonstrated _____ bacteria.

6. Mr. Manion complained to the doctor about that he couldn't keep his left upper eyelid from sagging. His doctor told him that he had a neurological problem called Horner syndrome, characterized by_____ of his eyelid.

7. After 6 weeks in a cast to set her broken arm, Jill's arm muscles were smaller and weaker. They had _____. Her physician recommended physical therapy to strengthen her arm.

8. Ms. Brody was diagnosed with breast cancer. The first phase of her treatment included a _____ to remove her breast and the tumor. Following the surgery, her doctors recommended chemotherapy with drugs such as Adriamycin and Taxol.

9. At the age of 29, Kevin's facial features became coarser, his hands and tongue enlarged. After a head CT scan, doctor diagnosed him with _____, a slowly

progressive endocrine condition involving the pituitary gland.

10. Each winter, when cold and flu season started, Daisy used to develop _____ _____. Her doctor prescribed antibiotics and respiratory therapy to help her recover.

11. After _____ on her knee, Ellen had swelling and inflammation near the small incisions. Dr. Nicholas assured her that this was a common side effect of the surgery that would resolve spontaneously.

12. David enjoyed lifting weights, but recently noticed a bulging in his right groin. He visited his doctor, who made the diagnosis of _____ and recommended surgical repair.

13. Under the microscope, Dr. Vance could see grape-like clusters of bacteria called streptococci. He made the diagnosis of _____ and antibiotics were started.

14. While ice skating, Natalie fell and landed on her buttocks. She had persistent _____ pain for a few weeks but no broken bone on X-ray examination.

15. When a proctologist examines a patient's anus, the patients should be in _____ _____position.

Section D   Writing

Health Record or Medical Records

The evolution of health records parallels advancements in medicine. The first incorporated hospital in the United States, Pennsylvania Hospital, was established in 1752. Benjamin Franklin served as the secretary for the hospital and recorded each patient's name, address, disorder, date of admission, and date of discharge. Massachusetts General Hospital in Boston has the distinction of having a complete medical record on each patient since 1821.

Today, technology affects all aspects of health care, and the health record is no exception. Hospitals and practitioners are moving from a paper-based record to an electronic health record. Whether paper-based or electronic, the health record is the link connecting all of health care. The health record is a valuable tool used by all entities involved in providing patient care, including practitioners, hospital, patient and family, and third-party payers.

In some settings, the health record is called the medical record, but the more updated term is health record. In this section we will provide an overview of the purpose, maintenance, and content of the health record.

1. Overview of the Health Record

The health record, whether paper-based or in electronic format, should contain sufficient information to justify the patient's diagnosis, treatment, and services rendered. Documentation in the record should explain the patient's progress including the response to therapy, medication or care rendered. Health records play the following roles in supporting the health-care industry.

- Serve as a communication tool that facilitates ongoing care and treatment of the patient.
- Justify reimbursement for hospitals and other health-care practitioners.
- Serve as legal document describing the health-care provided.
- Serve as a resource for research and education.
- Support clinical decision making.
- Provide information for evaluating the quality of care provided.
- Serve as a source of data for outcomes research.

2. Maintaining a Health Record

Health records are kept in one of three formats: paper format, electronic format, or a combination of both formats, known as a hybrid health record. Health records are maintained by all entities that provide health care to patients. Physicians, dentists, chiropractors, podiatrists, optometrists, nurses, physical therapists, occupational therapists, hospitals, urgent care centers, rehabilitation centers, skilled nursing facilities, residential facilities, emergency care facilities, home health-care agencies, behavioral health facilities, and correctional facilities are required to maintain a health record for each patient. Documentation requirements and the type of record maintained vary according to the type of facility and provider. Documented medical information links all aspects of the health-care delivery system; so, all health-care providers must document information to meet the needs of the patient and to comply with the laws and regulatory standards.

Maintaining a health record for patient encounters and documenting the care provided are mandatory. Over the decades, health-care has become increasingly complex resulting in the need to have documentation that is accurate, timely, and legible. Regulatory agencies such as the Joint Commission, the Commission on Accreditation of Rehabilitation Facilities (CARF), the Accreditation Association for Ambulatory health-care (AAAHC), the American Osteopathic Association (AOA), the National Committee on Quality Assurance (NCQA), and the American Accreditation health-care Commission (AAHC) are just a few of the accrediting agencies that have standards for health records and documentation. Attaining accreditation signifies that the institution has made a commitment to having high standards for performance improvement and quality improvement.

The federal government became more involved in health care in 1965 with the establishment of the Social Security Act, of which Medicare was a component. Medicare is a health insurance program for persons over the age of 65, persons under the age of 65 with certain disabilities, and individuals with end-stage renal disease requiring dialysis or a kidney transplant. Standards for health record content and documentation for federal patients are established by the Centers for Medicare & Medicaid Services (CMS), a division of the federal Department of Health and Human Services.

The health record must contain information to justify admission and continued hospitalization or outpatient ambulatory care, support the diagnosis, and describe patient's progress and response to medications/treatment and service.

Periodic reviews of health records by the state survey agency occur to ensure compliance with Medicare Conditions of Participation. Failure to demonstrate compliance could negatively impact reimbursement the provider and the health-care facility.

States also have specific documentation requirements as part of their licensure process. These regulations usually are under the direction of the state Department of Health. Failure to comply with the regulations could result in closure of the health-care facility.

3. Ensuring Quality Documentation in the Health Record

The therapist providing the care is responsible for making high-quality entries into the patient's health record. These entries must be timely, legible, and authenticated in accordance with the rules and regulations specified by the institutions in which the therapist works. Therapists will need to adhere to the documentation guidelines for their own profession. The following are documentation guidelines that all health-care providers should follow.

(1) All entries in the health record must be dated and signed with your name and professional designation to identify the author of the entry.

(2) Entries in the health record by graduates pending licensure or students in a physical therapy or physical therapist assistant program must be authenticated by a licensed physical therapist or physical therapist assistant when allowed by law.

(3) Entries in the health record cannot be erased or deleted. Corrections in a paper record are made by drawing one line through the error, leaving the incorrect material legible. The error should be initialed and dated so that it is obvious that it is a corrected mistake. If using an electronic health record system, use the appropriate procedure for indicating that a change was made without deletion in the original health record. The specific procedure for this will vary depending on the electronic health record program you are utilizing at your facility.

(4) All entries in the paper health record should always be made in black ink. Colors such as red, green, purple, and pink do not copy or scan well.

(5) Blank spaces should not be left in any documentation. Record an "X" in the blank area to prevent the insertion of additional information that would be out of date or out of sequence.

(6) All blanks on consent forms should be completed.

4. Location Information in the Paper Health Record

The health record is a repository of data. Locating information in the paper record can be challenging. This section provides an overview of the contents of the patient's health record to assist the therapist in pinpointing meaningful information.

The health record contains two types of data: administrative and clinical. Regulatory agencies or professional organizations do not mandate a specific form. Form design is the discretion of the health-care organization or health-care provider if working in private practice.

(1) Administrative Section

Administrative data include the patient's demographic information, such as name, address, date of birth, next of kin, payment source, billing or accounting number, and patient identification number, which is also called a health record number.

Demographic information is collected at the time of registration and recorded on a face sheet or top sheet of the health record. Facilities using a computer-based admission and discharge system will print out the demographic information on the face sheet or top sheet if the record is in a paper format.

At least two different pieces of demographic information must appear on each page of a patient's health record (paper format): the patient's name and the record number. Therapists should verify that they are making entries in the correct health record prior to making the entry.

Consent to release information, acknowledgment of patient rights, HIPAA acknowledgment, advance directives, consent to special procedures, property and valuables lists, and birth and death certificates are all considered administrative content.

(2) Clinical Section

Clinical content includes information related to the patient's condition, treatment, and progress. Clinical data make up most of the health record. Therapist must know each of the components of the clinical portion of the health record to be able to find the information needed for patient care.

(3) Health History

The health history and review of systems is the basis for formulating the provisional diagnosis and establishing a treatment plan. Contents of the history are somewhat subjective, since much of the information is provided by the patient or the patient's representative. Components of the health history include the following.

Chief complaint (CC): Stated in the patient's own words and explains why the patient is seeking treatment. Example: "My throat hurts."

History of present illness (HPI): Describes the duration, location, clinical signs and reason (cause) for the current condition, if known.

History of past illness: Documents any relevant childhood illness, previous surgeries, injuries, or illnesses that might have a bearing on the current condition. Allergies and drug sensitivities are also documented in the history of past illness.

Social history: Addresses habits, living conditions, occupation, material status, psychosocial needs, alcohol consumption, drug use, and tobacco use.

Family History: Documents conditions considered genetic or conditions of family members that might have relevance to the case such as diabetes, cardiovascular disease, or cancer.

Review of system (ROS): Asks questions that derive information that the patient might not have provided. All systems in the body are inventoried. Information in this section is not to be confused with the results of the physical examination as performed by the medical practitioner.

(4) Physical Examination

The physical examination provides objective data on the patient's condition. All body systems are included in the physical examination. There should be information in the record that addresses all the body systems with special emphasis on the areas that are pertinent to the Chief Complaint and the Review of systems. A clinical impression and course of action, based on the medical history and physical examination, conclude the history and physical. The therapist will find the history and physical examination beneficial in obtaining sufficient information to assist in patient care.

(5) Interdisciplinary Care Plan

The Interdisciplinary Care Plan lays the foundation for the care provided to the patient. Each profession associated with the patient contributes to the Interdisciplinary Care Plan, which includes an assessment of the patient, statement of desired goals for the patient, strategies on attaining the goals, and a periodic assessment of progress made toward achieving at scheduled intervals and revised as needed.

(6) Physician or Practitioner Orders

The Joint Commission defines a licensed independent practitioner as "any individual permitted by law and by the organization to provide care, treatment, and services without direction or supervision". As a therapist, it is important to determine your level of authority in writing orders by checking the facility's policies and procedures, as well as the bylaws, rules, regulation of the medical staff and state law.

Orders communicate the type of treatment and diagnostic procedure(s) the practitioner wants for the patient to carry out the care plan. Orders can be verbal or written. Verbal orders must be authenticated in accordance with state and federal regulation; bylaws, rules, and regulations of the medical staff; and regulatory agencies. Use of standing orders is discouraged because not all of the actions on the standing order may be medically necessary for the patient.

(7) Progress notes and patient/client management notes

Notes are interval statements that relate to observations about the patient's progress and response to treatment from the perspective of the professional. Although the frequency of a patient's treatment may vary, a note is required for every treatment attempt and for treatments that are provided. For every treatment provided, documentation should include what was done including frequency, intensity, and duration as appropriate, equipment used or provided, changes in the treatment plan, reaction to the treatment, and communication with the patient/family or other health-care providers.

In addition to dating and authenticating your progress/re-evaluation note, some facilities require that you provide a start and stop time documenting when you were with the patient. This will be important when billing for services rendered to the patient. Remember: Write your professional credentials after your signature.

(8) Consultation

A consultation report contains an opinion about a patient's condition by a practitioner other than the attending physician. It is important for the consultant to document his or her opinion based on a review of the patient record, examination of the patient, and conference with the attending physician. Consultants address their specialty area only.

(9) Discharge Summary and Clinical Resume

For patients who have a health record available from a previous admission, the discharge summary or clinical resume summarizes the patient's course in the hospital or other care setting. This is a great place to find significant finding from examinations, laboratory tests, procedures, and therapies, along with how the patient responded. The patient's condition on discharge, physical activity, diet, medications, and follow-up care are included in the discharge summary.

Pertinent information can be found elsewhere in the health record including the operative report, pathology report, nursing notes, medication administration record, laboratory reports, radiology and imaging reports, radiation therapy, and notes from therapists such as speech-language pathology, occupational therapy, physical therapy, respiratory therapy, and dietetics.

Remember, the health record is a communication tool. Although abbreviations, acronyms, and symbols save time when documenting, they can be misinterpreted by others, placing the patient at risk. If your facility has an approved abbreviation list, be sure to use only those abbreviations exactly as they appear in the approved list. The Joint commission has a list of abbreviations that are not to be used in the health record. The list can be accessed at jointcommission.org.

5. The Electronic Health Record

Health-care facilities are transitioning from a paper record to one that is computer-based, or electronic. Two terms used interchangeably are electronic medical record (EMR) and electronic health record (EHR). Even though the terms sound the same, there is a difference. The EMR came on the scene first. It made sense to use EMR because health-care was computerizing the "medical" aspect of patient care for the primary purpose of diagnosis and treatment.

The EHR supports patient care by capturing data to support the overall "health"of the patient-mind, body, and spirit. It is a repository for all the patient data collected from components of the electronic systems, such as computerized physician order entry, laboratory, pharmacy, radiology, imaging, admissions, and transcription. The EHR provides the caregivers, the patient, and others with access to patient-specific information or information on a group of patients for research purposes. At this point, it is fair to say that health care is somewhere between EMR and EHR. The EHR for the United States will take about another 10 to 15 years. We have a lot of catching up to do with the rest of the world!

6. Summary

Information contained in the health record links all of health care. The value of the health record to the care providers and institution is only as good as the documentation in the record. Therapists must take the initiative to follow the documentation guidelines specified in the rules and regulations where they work and to make timely entries in the health record. The EMR/EHR is being implemented throughout the health-care industry.

Exercise for health record

1. What kinds of roles do health records play in supporting the health-care industry ?
2. What kinds of documentation guidelines should all health-care providers follow ?

Section E   Spoken English

Role play

Directions: A patient got headache, on and off for about 2 weeks, and he went to clinic for help. 2 students work in pairs to demonstrate the conversation, one plays the role of doctor, the other of patient.

Discussion

Directions: Work in groups and discuss with your partners, then answer the following questions with detailed analysis.

A 13-year-old male presents to the Emergency Department with a chief complaint of sore throat and fever for the past 2 days. He reports that his younger sister has been ill for the past week with "the same thing". The patient has no other medical problems, takes on medications, and has no allergies. He denies any recent history of cough, rash, nausea, vomiting, or diarrhea. He denies any recent travel and has completed the full series of childhood immunizations.

On examination, the patient has a temperature of 38.5℃, a heart rate of 104 beats per minute, blood pressure 118/64 mmHg, a respiratory rate of 18 breaths per minute, and an oxygen saturation of 99% on room air. Oto-Rhino-Laryngogical (head, ears, eyes, nose, throat) exam reveals erythema of the posterior oropharynx with tonsillar exudates, but no uvular deviation or significant tonsillar swelling. Neck exam reveals mild tenderness of anterior lymph nodes. His neck is supple. The chest and cardiovascular exams are unremarkable, and his abdomen is non-tender with normal bowel sounds and no hepatosplenomegaly. His skin is without rash.

1. What is the most likely diagnosis?
2. What is your next step?
3. What are potential complications?

Chapter 2

Cardiovascular System

Section A　Focus Listening

Conversation

Listen to the dialogue and fill in the blanks with proper words.

D=doctor P=patient

D: What seems to be the problem at the moment?

P: I have dyspnea, chest pain and sometimes syncope.

D: Well, can you tell me how long you have had difficulty breathing?

P: It's a long story. Doctor, it has come and gone about two years.

D: When did the dyspnea attack, in the daytime or at night?

P: It often happens at night, doctor, but it's getting worse in the recent two weeks, you know, the dyspnea often wakes me up, and I have to sit upright and couldn't lie flat in bed.

D: Oh, _____ nocturnal dyspnea. And can you describe what the pain feels like?

P: Err..., it's just like pressure and heaviness on the chest.

D: Can you show me with your finger where the pain is?

P: Here, right behind the _____.

D: Is the pain just in that area or does it spread anywhere else?

P: It often radiates to right arm and little finger.

D: Does anything special bring it on?

P: It often occurs on physical exertion, excitement and _____ to cold, but eases after rest.

D: How long does the pain last each time?

P: It is often worse gradually, and lasts about 3-5 minutes and then disappears.

D: It is angina according to what you have described. And you said you had a _____?

P: Yes, syncope, it often occurs prior to or after exertion.

D: I need to listen to your chest, please undo your shirt.

P: OK.

D: Take a deep breath please, and hold on … a loud, rasping, crescendo- decrescendo systolic murmur along the right sternal border.

P: Please tell me what disease I got, doctor.

D: Don't worry about it, but you need to have _____ and ECG examination right away.

New Words & Expressions

dyspnea 呼吸困难   syncope 晕厥
paroxysmal 阵发性的   crescendo 声音渐强
nocturnal 夜间的   decrescendo 声音渐弱
sternum 胸骨   systolic 收缩期的
exertion 努力；费力   ultrasound 超声波
angina 心绞痛

Passage

Answer the questions after listening to the passage.

1. Which part of the heart is damaged due to the decreased blood supply?

A. Epicardium.   B. Myocardium.

C. Endocardium.   D. All of the above.

2. What does the term Angina refer to?

A. Abdominal pain.   B. Body pain.

C. Pain in the heart.   D. Pain in the head.

3. What is the name of the blood vessel that supply blood to the heart?

A. Hepatic artery.   B. Renal artery.

C. Coronary artery.   D. Cerebral artery.

4. What are the common risk factors for heart disease?

A. Healthy diet.   B. Smoking.

C. Alcohol consumption.   D. Both B and C.

5. What is the name of the substance in the blood that blocks blood vessels?

A. Fatty acid.   B. Cholesterol.

C. Glucose.   D. Proteins.

Section B   Reading Comprehension

Text

A 19-year-old white male presents to the emergency department (ED) in Connecticut after an episode of shortness of breath and syncope while at home. He reports having experienced recurrent episodes of palpitations and fatigue in the week before presentation. Yesterday, the patient sought medical attention for these symptoms at his pediatrician's office. An electrocardiogram (ECG) was performed, but it was normal; the patient was sent home wearing a Holter monitor (also known as an ambulatory electrocardiography device). Today, while mowing the lawn, the patient again felt a sudden onset of palpitations, accompanied by shortness of breath and lightheadedness. He went inside the house, where he suddenly "passed out" (according to the patient's girlfriend). The girlfriend also stated that he was unresponsive for a couple of minutes and that the patient exhibited no seizure like activity or incontinence. She noted that he was "pretty much himself" once he regained consciousness. He was then brought by ambulance to the ED; a rhythm strip was acquired en route. Prophylactic transcutaneous pacer pads were placed by the emergency medical services (EMS) team.

In the ED, the patient describes his palpitations as irregular, forceful beats, with a sensation of a racing heart. They occur spontaneously, without any clear inciting factors. He denies having any chest pain or shortness of breath at the time of questioning in the ED. He has not experienced any similar events prior to these, and he is usually active and athletic. The patient denies having any recent fevers, upper respiratory infections, cough, or sore throat. He denies having any recent headaches, neck stiffness, tinnitus, vertigo, or focal neurologic deficits. He also denies experiencing any bleeding (e.g., no hematochezia or melena). The patient has been eating a regular diet and has not had any weight loss recently. His past medical history is only significant for a cervical spine fracture secondary to a diving accident that occurred 3 years ago. He has no residual deficits or physical limitations. The patient is otherwise healthy, with no known cardiac, neurologic, or pulmonary disease. He has no known family history of sudden death or premature cardiac disease. He does not take any regular medications, and he denies any drug abuse, tobacco use, or alcohol consumption. The Holter monitor had been removed before he began to mow the lawn; therefore, no results were available to ED staff.

On physical examination, the patient appears to be in no acute distress, but he is noted to have moderate anxiety. He is nontoxic-appearing and alert. His vital signs include a temperature of 96.7℉ (35.9℃), a pulse rate between 40-120 bpm, a respiratory rate of 16 breaths/min, and a blood pressure of 102/46 mmHg. His oxygen saturation is 96% while breathing room air. His head and neck examination are unremarkable. No jugular venous distention or carotid bruits are noted. His lungs are clear to auscultation bilaterally. His cardiac examination reveals an irregular, tachycardic rhythm. There is no discernible murmur with or without Valsalva maneuvers or hand clenching. His abdomen is soft, non-tender, and non-distended. No clubbing, cyanosis, or edema is noted in his extremities. His neurologic examination is normal. On skin examination, multiple, bilateral macular erythematous lesions with large central pallor are noted on his thighs.

An ECG is obtained.

New Words & Expressions

episode [ˈepɪsəʊd] *n.* something that take place 发作

syncope [ˈsɪŋkəpi] *n.* loss of consciousness resulting from insufficient blood flow to the brain 晕厥

electrocardiography [elektrəʊˈkɑːdɪəʊɡrəfi] *n.* 心电描记法

lightheadedness *n.* mentally disoriented, dizzy 眩晕

pass out to become unconscious 昏倒，失去知觉

seizure [ˈsiːʒər] *n.* sudden occurrence (or recurrence) of a disease 发作

incontinence [ɪnˈkɒntɪnəns] *n.* inability of the body to control the evacuative functions of urination or defecation 大小便失禁

pretty much most completely 几乎全部

en route [en ruːt] on the way 在途中

prophylactic [ˌprɒfɪˈlæktɪk] *a.* guarding from or preventing the spread or occurrence of disease or infection 预防疾病的

transcutaneous [ˌtrænzkjʊˈteniəs] *a.* passing, entering, or made by penetration through the skin 经皮（性）的；由皮的

incite [ɪnˈsaɪt] *v.* to move on, stir on, urge on 激励；激起

tinnitus [ˈtɪnɪtəs] *n.* a ringing or booming sensation in one or both ears; a symptom of an ear infection or Meniere's disease 耳鸣

hematochezia [hɛmətəˈkiziə] *v.* bright red blood is found in the feces 便血

melena [məˈliːnə] *n.* abnormally dark tarry feces containing blood (usually from gastrointestinal bleeding) 黑粪症

saturation [ˌsætʃəˈreɪʃ(ə)n] *n.* the act of saturating : the state of being saturated 饱和

macular [ˈmækjʊlə] *n.* of macula 斑疹的，斑的

erythematous [ˌerɪˈθiːmətəs] *a.* abnormal redness of the skin due to capillary congestion 红斑的

Exercise

Decide whether the following statements are true(T) or false(F) according to the passage.

_____1. The 19-year-old white male patient sought medical attention for his symptoms at his attending physician's office.

_____2. The patient's girlfriend states that he just lost consciousness for several minutes and didn't have any seizure like activity or incontinence.

_____3. The patient hasn't had any experience of chest pain or shortness of breath prior to this time because he doesn't have the habit of doing exercises.

_____4. The Holter monitor had been removed before the patient began to mow the lawn; Therefore, ED staff couldn't get any available results.

_____5.The patient's vital signs include a temperature of 96.7°F (35.9°C), a pulse rate between 80-120 bpm, and a blood pressure of 102/46 mmHg on physical examination.

Answer the following questions according to the passage.

1.What is the most likely diagnosis according to symptoms and lab findings such as multiple, bilateral macular erythematous lesions with large central pallor are noted on his thighs?

_____

2.What first-line antibiotics will be used to treat the patient?

_____

Use the appropriate form of the words or phrases in the box to complete the following sentences.

respiratory	palpitation	syncope	cyanosis	auscultation
erythematous	distention	prophylactic	fracture	thigh
pulmonary	tinnitus	cardiac		

1. Inspection, _____ and olfaction, inquiry and pulse-taking and palpation are the four diagnostic methods to understand the pathological conditions.

2. They suspect he is suffering from a _____ embolism, basically a blood clot in an artery of the lung that could prove fatal.

3. Shakiness, cold sweating, _____, and hunger sensation are some of the

initial symptoms of hypoglycemia which result from adrenergic effect.

4. A gastric tube is indicated to reduce stomach _____ and decrease the risk of aspiration.

5. Similarly, most physicians advocate giving _____ platelet transfusions to reduce the likelihood of bleeding.

6. In these patients, the virus directly infects the lung, causing severe _____ failure.

7. All patients didn't appear the symptoms of vascular and nerve injury and the situation of _____ fixation.

8. Zipes said if doctors can figure out how Clark's heart healed itself and develop a treatment from that mechanism, many other _____ patients could benefit.

9. _____ is the major indication that there is a problem with many newborn babies.

10. A 27-year-old female presented with several annular plaques on the upper back for one month. Other dermatologic findings revealed _____ plagues with mild scaling on the scalp.

Translation

A. Translate the following expressions into English.

1. 反复发作的心悸　　　　　　2. 动态心电描记法装置
3. 恢复意识　　　　　　　　　4. 局灶性神经功能缺损
5. 猝死家族史　　　　　　　　6. 体格检查
7. 脉搏　　　　　　　　　　　8. 血压

B. Translate the following sentences or expressions into Chinese.

1. In the ED, the patient describes his palpitations as irregular, forceful beats, with a sensation of a racing heart, which occur spontaneously, without any clear inciting factors.

2. There is no discernible murmur with or without Valsalva maneuvers or hand clenching.

3. He does not take any regular medications, and he denies any drug abuse, tobacco use, or alcohol consumption.

4. The patient has been eating a regular diet and has not had any recent weight loss.

5. Today, while mowing the lawn, the patient again felt a sudden onset of palpitations, accompanied by shortness of breath and lightheadedness.

Section C   Vocabulary (Terminology)

1. 心 heart, cor

Combining form	Meaning	Terminology	Terminology meaning
cardio-	heart	cardiology	the study of the heart and its action and diseases 心脏病学
corono-	heart	coronary	of, relating to, or being the coronary arteries or veins of the heart; broadly: of or relating to the heart 冠状动脉的，心脏的

2. 心房 atrium

Combining form	Meaning	Terminology	Terminology meaning
atrio-	atrium, upper heart chamber	atrioventricular	of, relating to, or located between an atrium and ventricle of the heart 房室的

3. 心室 ventricle

Combining form	Meaning	Terminology	Terminology meaning
ventriculo-	ventricle, lower heart chamber	ventricular	of, relating to, or being a ventricle

4. 瓣膜 valve

Combining form	Meaning	Terminology	Terminology meaning
valvo-	valve	valvulitis	inflammation of a valve especially of the heart 心脏瓣膜炎
-cuspid	of cuspid	bicuspid	having or ending in two points 二尖瓣

5. vessel 血管

Combining form	Meaning	Terminology	Terminology meaning
vaso-	vessel	vasoconstriction	narrowing of the lumen of blood vessels 血管收缩
vasculo-	vessel	vascular	supplied with or made up of such channels and especially blood vessels 脉管的，血管的
angio-	vessel	angiogram	a radiograph made by angiography 血管造影片

6. 动脉 artery

Combining form	Meaning	Terminology	Terminology meaning
arterio-artero-	artery	arteriosclerosis	a chronic disease characterized by abnormal thickening and hardening of the arterial walls with resulting loss of elasticity 动脉硬化症

7. 静脉 vein

Combining form	Meaning	Terminology	Terminology meaning
veno-	vein	venous	of, relating to, or full of veins 静脉的
veni-	vein	venipuncture	surgical puncture of a vein especially for the withdrawal of blood or for intravenous medication 静脉穿刺
phlebo-	vein	thrombophlebitis	inflammation of a vein with formation of a thrombus 血栓性静脉炎

8. 主动脉 aorta

Combining form	Meaning	Terminology	Terminology meaning
aorto-	aorta	aortic	of or relating with aorta 主动脉的

9. 毛细血管 capillary

Combining form	Meaning	Terminology	Terminology meaning
capillario-	capillary	capillarity	the action by which the surface of a liquid where it is in contact with a solid (as in a capillary tube) is elevated or depressed depending on the relative attraction of the molecules of the liquid for each other and for those of the solid 毛细管作用

10. 脉 pulse

Combining form	Meaning	Terminology	Terminology meaning
sphygmo-	pulse	sphygmomanometer	an instrument for measuring blood pressure and especially arterial blood pressure 血压计

11. 血 blood

Combining form	Meaning	Terminology	Terminology meaning
hemo-	blood	hemolysis	lysis of red blood cells with liberation of hemoglobin 溶血现象, 血细胞溶解
hemato-	blood	hematocrit	the ratio of the volume of red blood cells to the total volume of blood as determined by separation of red blood cells from the plasma usually by centrifugation 血细胞比容, 红细胞压积

12. 脂肪变性, 动脉粥样硬化 athero-

Combining form	Meaning	Terminology	Terminology meaning
athero-	yellowish plaque, fatty substance	atheroma	fatty degeneration of the inner coat of the arteries 动脉粥样化

13. 臂 arm

Combining form	Meaning	Terminology	Terminology meaning
brachi/o-	arm	brachial artery	臂动脉

14. 胆固醇 cholesterol

Combining form	Meaning	Terminology	Terminology meaning
cholesterol/o	cholesterol (substance)	hypercholesterolemia	the presence of excess cholesterol in the blood 高胆固醇血症

15. 蓝，青紫 cyan/o

Combining form	Meaning	Terminology	Terminology meaning
cyan/o	blue	cyanosis	a bluish or purplish discoloration (as of skin) due to deficient oxygenation of the blood 发绀

16. 粘液 myx/o

Combining form	Meaning	Terminology	Terminology meaning
myx/o-	mucus	myxoma	a benign tumor derived from connective tissue, with cells embedded in soft mucoid stromal tissue, these tumor occur most frequently in the left atrium 黏液瘤

17. 氧 oxygen, ox/o–

Combining form	Meaning	Terminology	Terminology meaning
ox/o	oxygen	hypoxia	a deficiency of oxygen reaching the tissues of the body 组织缺氧

18. 心包 pericardium

Combining form	Meaning	Terminology	Terminology meaning
pericardi/o	pericardium	pericardiocentesis	surgical puncture to remove fluid 心包穿刺术

19. 胸 stetho–

Combining form	Meaning	Terminology	Terminology meaning
stetho-	chest	stethoscope	a medical instrument for detecting sounds produced in the body that are conveyed to the ears of the listener through rubber tubing connected with a piece placed upon the area to be examined 听诊器

Exercise

Match the following pathological condition or term with their meaning below.

stethoscope	cardiology	hypoxia	myxoma	cyanosis
hemolysis	capillarity	hematocrit	hypercholesterolemia	
venipuncture	angioma	sphygmomanometer		thrombophlebitis
coronary	valvulitis	atheroma	atrioventricular	vasoconstriction

_____1. The study of the heart and its action and diseases.

_____2. The ratio of the volume of red blood cells to the total volume of blood as determined by separation of red blood cells from the plasma usually by centrifugation.

_____3. Of, relating to, or located between an atrium and ventricle of the heart.

_____4. The action by which the surface of a liquid where it is in contact with a solid (as in a capillary tube) is elevated or depressed depending on the relative attraction of the molecules of the liquid for each other and for those of the solid.

_____5. The presence of excess cholesterol in the blood.

_____6. A medical instrument for detecting sounds produced in the body that are conveyed to the ears of the listener through rubber tubing connected with a piece placed upon the area to be examined.

_____7. A benign tumor derived from connective tissue, with cells embedded in soft mucoid stromal tissue, these tumors occur most frequently in the left atrium.

_____8. Lysis of red blood cells with liberation of hemoglobin.

_____9. An instrument for measuring blood pressure and especially arterial blood pressure.

_____10. Fatty degeneration of the inner coat of the arteries.

_____11. Inflammation of a vein with formation of a thrombus.

_____12. Narrowing of the lumen of blood vessels.

_____13. A tumor composed chiefly of blood vessels or lymph vessels.

_____14. Inflammation of a valve especially of the heart.

_____15. Surgical puncture of a vein especially for the withdrawal of blood or for intravenous medication.

_____16. A bluish or purplish discoloration (as of skin) due to deficient oxygenation of the blood.

_____17. A deficiency of oxygen reaching the tissues of the body.

_____18. Of, relating to, or being the coronary arteries or veins of the heart; broadly:

of or relating to the heart.

Choose the term that best completes the meaning of the sentence.

1. A 55-year-old male presented with chest choking, fatigue and lightheadedness for 4 months. He stated that the syncope suddenly presented and 5 minutes later he regained the consciousness, the heart rate was 40 beats/min. So what's the most likely diagnosis in ECG?

A. Sinus bradycardia.

B. Grade Ⅰ atrioventricular block.

C. Grade Ⅱ atrioventricular block.

D. Grade Ⅲ atrioventricular block.

2. A 58-year-old female with a history of hypertension for 10 years complained of intermittent chest pain and choking for 2 years which was diagnosed as hypertension and atherosclerotic heart diseases. He stated he was treated by propranolol hydrochloride 10mg, t.i.d. However, he suddenly had chest choking, shortness of breath with foamy sputum. On physical examination: orthopnea, hear rate 110 beats/min, moist rales heard on the bottom of both lungs, edema not found in both limbs. What's the most likely diagnosis?

A. Acute bronchopneumonia.

B. Acute left heart failure.

C. Heart failure.

D. Acute myocardial infarction.

3. A 26-year-old unmarried female with a history of tuberculosis complained of distending pain in abdomen and fatigue, shortness of breath after exertion. On physical examination: BP: 90/75mmHg, apical heart beats not easily palpable. Heart not enlarged, heart rate 120 beats/min with atrial fibrillation rhythm with engorgement of jugular veins which is distinct on inhalation, abdomen soft, the liver palpable 3cm below the coastal margin, shifting dullness positive, slight edema found in both lower limbs, chest fluoroscopy reveals no blood stasis found in both lungs with dilation of superior vena cava, small arch of aorta and normal cardiac shadow. ECG shows low voltage in QRS waves, depression of T wave and inverted T wave present. What's the major mechanism of clinical manifestations mentioned above?

A. Decreased cardiac contraction.

B. The blockage of ventricular filling due to pericardium stenosis.

C. Over-afterload of the heart.

D. Over-preload of the heart.

4. Ms. Hu, aged 45, complained of intermittent sudden onset of headache, dizziness, perspiration and dyspnea for 2 years, he stated that the blood pressure is 200/120 mmHg on episode, the symptoms spontaneous disappear in 2 hours, the blood decrease to normal limits. What's the most likely diagnosis?

A. Hypertensive crisis.

B. Pheochromocytoma.

C. Renal artery stenosis.

D. Hypertension.

5. A 65-year-old retired cadre with a history of recurrent chest choking and palpitation for 30 years was admitted to hospital complaining of sharp retrosternal pain 12 hours. He had previously been well, has a past medical history of hypercholesterolemia, and a 30-pack-month history of smoking. On examination, he appears uncomfortable and diaphoretic with a heart rate of 95 beats/min, a blood pressure of 166/102 mmHg, and a respiratory rate of 22 breaths/min with an oxygen saturation of 96% on room air, the jugular venous pressure appears normal. Auscultation of the chest reveals clear lung fields, and a regular heart rate with a S4 gallop and no murmur or rubs. A chest shows clear lungs and a normal cardiac silhouette. The ECG is shown in Figure 1. So, what's the most likely diagnosis?

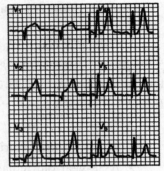

Figure 1 Image of the patient's ECG

A. Hypertension.　　　　　　　B. Acute myocardial infarction.

C. Aortic dissection.　　　　　　D. Acute pericarditis.

6. A 21-year-old female was admitted to hospital complaining of recurrent arthralgia for 5 years and palpitation and shortness of breath after exertion for 1 day. On physical examination: pear-shaped heart contours, heart rate 88 beats/min with regular rhythm, a rumbling diastolic murmur heard over apex, P2 accentuated, Hb 88g/L. What's the diagnosis?

A. Left atrial myxoma.

B. Anemia.

C. Coronary heart disease.

D. Rheumatic heart disease, mitral stenosis.

7. A 25-year-old male was admitted to hospital complaining of shortness of breath and edema of lower limbs for 2 months. On examination: heart enlarged, grade II ～ III blowing systolic murmur heard in apical region, trace moist rales heard in both lungs, the liver enlarged, edema of lower limbs. Ultrasound examination shows significantly enlarged both left atrium and ventricle. The probably diagnosis is _____.

A. coronary heart disease.

B. rheumatic heart disease with mitral incompetence.

C. acute viral myocarditis.

D. dilated cardiomyopathy.

8. A 24-year-old male presented your office complaining of tachypnea and distending abdomen for 2 months, on examination: BP 90/75mmHg, engorgement of jugular vein, the heart contours enlarged to both sides, heart rate 120 beats/min with regular rhythm, weak heart sound, the liver palpable 3 fingers below the coastal margin, ascites sign positive,

edema in both lower limbs. What's the most likely diagnosis?

A. Liver cirrhosis.

B. Constrictive pericarditis.

C. Acute pericarditis with effusion.

D. Rheumatic heart disease, heart failure.

9. Ms. Peng, 76-year-old, had recurrent episode of syncope with jerk for past 2 days. She denied having history of chest pain, shortness of breath, cyanosis and edema of lower limbs. On examination: BP 180/80mmHg, P 40/min with regular rhythm, fluctuated intensity of S1 heard in the apical region, grade Ⅱ ejection heart murmur heard in bottom of heart. What's the most possible cause resulting in recurrent syncope with jerk?

A. Hypertensive encephalopathy.

B. Sinus bradycardia with premature ventricular contraction.

C. Grade I atrioventricular block.

D. Complete atrioventricular block.

10. A 66-year-old male was admitted to hospital complaining persistent sharp chest pain with shortness of breath unable to lie down. On physical examination: the heart enlarged leftward, heart rate 140 beats/min with regular rhythm, decreased S1, fine moist rales and trace wheezing heard in both lungs, ECG shows: QR waves present in V1~V6, ST segment are significantly elevated. Which of the following medication is not proper?

A. Cedilanid drop.   B. Nitroglycerin drop.

C. Morphine drop.   D. Beta blockers.

Section D   Writing

Medical records

Mrs. Jane Doe

Registration 12345

432 Maple Avenue

Babylon, California Tel (123) 456-7899

August 31, 1982 2:00 P.M.

CC (Chief Complaint): This 45-year-old married mother has had episodic right upper quadrant"knife-like"pain for the past 2 days.

HPI (History of Present Illness): Mrs. Doe was in her usual good state of health until 2 days ago (August 29) when having just finished a pork-chop dinner, she had severe "knife-like" pain in the right upper quadrant of her abdomen, radiating to her epigastrium.

She concurrently felt "sick to her stomach" (without vomiting), sweaty, and faint (without loss of consciousness). She immediately lay down on her bed and felt better after a minute. The severe pain grew rapidly less, as did the nausea, but she had a "dull ache" in her right upper quadrant for several hours. She took no medication. Position did not affect the pain. She felt well enough after an hour to clean up the dinner table and slept well that night. She has had two subsequent"attacks", the first at lunch yesterday (August 30) following hamburger and French fries. The most recent episode was at breakfast today after two slices of bacon.

She's had no fever, chills, vomiting, or diarrhea. She denies past history of similar episodes. She has no current or past history of jaundice, white stools, dark urine, or change in bowel habits. She is unaware of a history of anemia (other than mild "low blood" associated with her first pregnancy). She has not had tarry or black stools, hematemesis, burning abdominal pain or other "indigestion", kidney stones, polyuria or hematuria, hepatitis, or foreign travel. She has had no cough, shortness of breath, or pleurisy. She has no calf pain. She regularly examines her breasts and has noted no masses. There is a history of breast cancer in her mother. She has no known heart disease. She denies trauma to her chest, back, or legs. Her menses have been normal. She takes no regular medications and specifically denies the use of antacids, aspirin, clofibrate (Atromid), or alcohol. She currently feels quite well.

PMH (Past Medical History):

Childhood illness: Mumps and chickenpox as child. No measles, rheumatic fever, scarlet fever.

Adult illness: None significant. Hospitalized only for childbirth (Soma Hospital, Babylon-1961 and 1963)

Trauma: Fractured left clavicle as child. No sequelae.

Surgery: Tonsillectomy as child of 6 (Soma Hospital). Episiotomy with each childbirth.

Allergies: Penicillin-urticarial rash without wheezing, stridor, (last dose 1976, at which time reaction occurred).

Medications: None at present. Has taken occasional aspirin for headache in past.

Travel: Never outside California.

Habits: Has never smoked tobacco or cannabis. Occasionally dinner wine (none in past 2 weeks). No illicit drugs. Regular diet, 3 meals a day.

Immunizations: Does not remember childhood shots other than oral polio vaccine in early 1950s. Last tetanus shot 7 years ago.

Family History: No family history of renal disease, liver disease, hypertension, anemia, tuberculosis.

Social History: Mrs. Doe was born and raised in Babylon, where she married her current husband after her graduation from high school in 1955. She worked as a secretary in his construction firm until their first child was born in 1961. She remained at home to raise her two sons, both of whom are college students (majoring in art and mathematics, respectively), and has recently returned to night school to gain college credits herself. She describes her life as full and her marriage as happy. Activities include housekeeping, gardening, and reading "romantic novels". Her husband's medical coverage extends to her, and she is not worried about money. She does admit to some unhappiness at not having gone to college as a young woman, but "is making up for it now". She is worried that her pain may represent an illness that will interfere with her studies, and she has "a test coming up next week". She is also fearful of cancer, as her mother has metastatic cancer of the breast, which is painful and emotionally draining on Mrs. Doe, who visits her in a nursing home every day.

Review of System:

General: See HPI. No weight changes.

Head: Occasional"stress"headache. No dizziness. "Faintness" with her recent attacks as described in HPI.

Eyes: last tested 1 year ago at 20/20. No blurring, double vision, pain, discharge.

Ears: No decreased hearing, tinnitus, pain. Otitis media once as child (right ear).

Nose: No epistaxis, sinusitis.

Throat and mouth: Teeth in good repair. Infrequent sore throats.

Chest: See HPI. No wheezing, hemoptysis, sputum. Chest X-ray normal on screening exam 1 year ago. Negative TB skin test 1 year ago.

Heart: No pain, palpitations, orthopnea, cyanosis, edema. No history hypertension.

GI (Gastrointestinal): see HPI.

GU (genitourinary): See HPI. No dysuria, frequency, urgency, incontinence. No history venereal disease or urinary tract infection.

Menstrual: Menarche age 13. Periods light flow for 3 days every 28 days and regular, with slight cramping on 1st day of flow. Last period normal, ended August 19, C2P2A0.

Neuromuscular: Faintness as in HPI, without syncope. No vertigo, dysesthesias(multiple sclerosis pain), seizures. No history emotional disease.

Physical Examination:

August 31, 1982

2:30 P.M.

General: Mrs. Doe is a slightly obese pleasant 45-year-old white woman who is somewhat anxious but in no acute distress.

Weight: 132lbs, Height: 5'6"

Vital Signs: T 99 ℉ orally, P85 regular, R12

BP R sitting: 140/90

L arm sitting: 148/92

L arm standing: 155/95

Skin: Warm and dry. No petechiae, purpura, excoriations (an abraded area where the skin is torn or worn off). Anicteric. Hair and nails normal. No cutaneous lesions or rashes.

Nodes: No cervical, supraclavicular, epitrochlear lymphadenopathy. 1 cm × 1cm, soft, non-tender, mobile node R axilla. Scattered shotty inguinal nodes bilaterally.

Head: Normocephalic, without trauma. No scars, tenderness, bruits.

Eyes: Conjunctivae normal. Slight scleral icterus bilaterally. Lids without lesions. Pupils equal, round, and react to light and accommodation. Vision equally normal (reads newspaper). Visual fields full to confrontation. Extraocular motions full, without strabismus or nystagmus. Fundus shows normal discs and vasculature. No arteriovenous nicking, silver-wiring, hemorrhage, or exudate.

Ears: External ears normal. Tympanic membranes normal bilaterally. Weber midline. Air conduction greater than bone bilaterally.

Nose: Nasal mucosa normal, without inflammation, obstruction, or polyps.

Mouth: Lips, buccal mucosa without lesions. Tongue well papillate, pink, midline. Teeth in good repair. Uvula midline. Oropharynx without inflammation or lesions.

Neck: Supple. Trachea midline. Thyroid not enlarged and without nodules. Jugular veins flat. Venous pulses normal. Carotid 4+ without bruits, normal pulse contour bilaterally.

Chest and lungs: Chest wall contour normal, with symmetrical full expansion, No rib tenderness to palpation. Tactile fremitus normal. Diaphragmatic excursion 5cm bilaterally. No percussion dullness. Lungs are clear to auscultation save for an isolated musical wheeze on forced expiration at the right base posteriorly. There is no egophony over this area. No rubs heard.

Heart: No visible lifts, PMI palpable 8 cm from the L sternal border in the 6th intercostal space. No palpable thrills, lifts, heaves. Rhythm regular, rate 80. S1 normal, S2 physiologically split. There is no S3 but a soft S4 at the apex. There is a 2/6 systolic ejection murmur at the L sternal border, without radiation. No rubs, no diastolic murmurs.

Breast: R breast slightly larger than L. No retractions, visible dimpling or skin changes. Nipples normal, everted. 2cm × 2cm cystic, mobile, non-tender mass without skin fixation in upper outer R breast. No nipple discharges.

Abdomen: Slightly protuberant. No scars or visible masses. Venous pattern normal. Bowel sounds normal. No hepatic or splenic rubs. No bruits. Liver is 15 cm to percussion and is 3cm below the right costal margin. Liver edge is smooth and tender to with positive Murphy's sign. No epigastric tenderness. Spleen and kidneys not palpable. No shifting dullness or fluid wave. No hernia.

Pelvic and rectal: External genitalia normal, including Bartholin's and Skeine's glands. Vaginal vault without lesions or discharge. Cervix parous, without lesions or discharge. Pap smear taken.

Bimanual: Fundus normal, in size & position. No tenderness. Ovaries and ligament felt and are without masses or tenderness.

Rectovaginal: Confirms bimanual.

Rectum: No anal lesions. Sphincter tone normal. No masses. Stool is clay -colored and for occult blood.

Extremities: Pulses fill and symmetrical, without bruits. Skin and hair are normal on extremities.

Pulse:

	carotid	Supra-clavicular	radial	brachial	Aorta	Femoral	DP	PT
$4+=N\dfrac{R}{L}$	4+	3+	4+	4+	0	4+	4+	4+
	4+	3+	4+	4+	0	4+	4+	4+

No clubbing, cyanosis, or edema. No swelling, redness, tenderness, limitation of movement of joints. No visible varicosities. No calf tenderness or cords. Muscle mass normal bilaterally.

Back: Slight cervical kyphosis. No spinal tenderness, CVA tenderness or sacral edema. Full range of motion spine.

Neurologic:

Mental status: Alert, oriented. Memory, judgment, mood normal.

Cranial nerves:

I -Not tested.

II -Pupils react to light. Reads Newspapers

III , IV , VI -NO strabismus. EOM normal.

VI -Corneal reflex intact.

VII -Face symmetrical.

VIII -Hearing normal.

IX , X -Uvula elevates symmetrically.

XI -Trapezius, sternomastoid normal.

XII -Tongue protrudes midline.

Cerebellar: Gait, finger-nose, and heel-shin normal.

Station and gait: Romberg negative; Heel-toe walk normal.

Motor: Muscle mass normal. Good strength in arm and legs.

Deep tendon reflexes: 2 + = NI.

No pathological reflexes.

Sensory: Normal to touch, pinpricks, vibration.

Laboratory Findings:

Hemogram: Hgb (hemoglobin)14.2, Hct (hematocrit) 46%, WBC 8500, Polyps 65, Bands 5, Monos (monocyte) 10, Lymphs (lymphocyte) 19, Eos (eosinophil) 1, Baso (basophil) 0. Peripheral smear: Normocytic, normochromic RBCs. No fragments, targets, nucleated RBC. WBC morphology normal. Platelets abundant on smear.

Urine: Clear, dark yellow. SG1.015. Dipstix neg. heme, protein, glucose, ketones. 3 + for bilirubin, pH = 6. Micro: 0-1 WBC, 0 RBC, no organisms per high-power field. No crystals, casts.

Serologics:

Electrolytes: Na: 140, K= 4.2, Cl: 100, Ca:10, P= 3.4, albumin= 4.0, Glob-3.5, SGOT:123, SGPT= 85, Alkaline Phosphatase= 210, Bilirubin total= 4.0, Bilirubin direct= 3.5, Serum amylase= 236, GI= 123, Cr= 1.0, BUN= 10

Chest X-ray: Bones normal, without blastic or lytic lesions. Heart shows slight straightening L heart border. Parenchyma clear except for slight linear atelectasis R base posteriorly (R lower lobe, basal seg). No evident effusion.

KUB: Bones normal. Psoas shadows seen. Nephrograms show normal size kidneys. Bowel gas normal. No evident ascites. Speckled calcification medial RUQ in area gallbladder.

ECG: Rate= 80, rhythm= sinus, PR= 0.15, QRS= 0.10, QT= 0.32, Axis= + 30. P waves normal. QRS normal. No T wave flattening or ST segment abnormalities. No LVH by voltage. Impression= normal ECG.

Impressions:

1. RUQ pain

a. R/O cholecystitis with cholelithiasis. This is supported by the historical relationship of RUQ sharp pains associated with fatty foods, scleral icterus, hepatomegaly, and + Murphy's sign, clay-colored stools, and laboratory finding of bilirubinuria, abnormal liver function studies with an obstructive pattern, hyperamylasemia, and calcification on KUB that might represent gallstones. The RLL atelectasis on chest film is not inconsistent with an intra-abdominal process.

b. R/O carcinomatosis of the liver. With her family history of breast cancer the breast mass and node on physical examination, this diagnosis must be considered. The episodicity of her pain, the lack of nodularity of the liver, and the absence of evident disease elsewhere makes this less likely.

c. R/O pulmonary embolism. Though unlikely, the RLL wheeze on P. E. and atelectasis on chest film could represent the site of lodgment of pulmonary embolism from the legs (for which there is no local evidence of phlebitis) or peripelvic (She has had 2 children) areas. The liver disease in this circumstance would represent congestive hepatopathy from transient right failure of pulmonary embolism.

d. R/O myocardial infarction or ischemia. This is very improbable with her history, but should be considered in light of her recent stress in classes and the association of her pain with eating. Her hypertension, though mild, could predispose her. In this circumstance, her liver disease would be transient congestive hepatopathy.

Although other diagnosis is possible (infective pneumonia, pancreatitis, peptic ulcer, infective or toxic hepatitis), there is little to support them in the history or physical examination.

Plan

1. RUQ pain

Plan: I will hospitalize her today and obtain an ECHO of her gall bladder and biliary tree. Should this prove nondiagnostic, I would proceed to prepare her for an oral cholecystogram.

I will ask the surgeon to see her today, should another attack occasion the need for emergency surgical intervention.

Serial physical examination, urine bilirubin testing, and serum liver function tests will allow monitoring of her process.

2. Right breast mass and axillary node with PH cancer of the breast

Although the cystic lesion of the breast probably does not represent a malignancy' her FH and deep concern are troublesome.

Plan: Mammography and probably biopsy of the mass are in order. These be done on this hospitalization.

3. Hypertension

Although this might be due to anxiety, the presence of the S_4 and the strengthening of left heart border on chest film suggest a fixed hypertension rather than labile one.

Plan: I will monitor her pressure in hospital. Should they remain elevated, salt restricted weight loss and probably diuretic therapy will be instituted.

4. Allergy to penicillin

Her urticaria response could presage anaphylaxis.

Plan: I will instruct the nurses to flag her chart as allergy to penicillin. On discharge, Mrs. Doe should obtain medic-alert to the effect that she is allergic to this drug.

5. Systolic heart murmur

This is probably a flow murmur.

Plan: Observe.

(signature)

I. H. Galen, M.D.

Section E   Spoken English

Role play

Directions: A patient got a heart problem, which comes and goes for about 2 years, and he went to clinic for help. Two students are selected to demonstrate the conversation, one plays the role of doctor, the other the patient.

Discussion

Directions: Work in groups and discuss with your partners, and then answer the following questions with detailed analysis.

MT, a 68-year-old white man, was brought to the emergency department by his wife after he experienced chest discomfort that did not resolve after 6 to 7 hours. He initially thought that his symptoms were due to indigestion and heartburn and was thus reluctant to seek medical help. His medical history is significant for hyperlipidemia (treated with atorvastatin 10 mg/d), mild hypertension (controlled on a salt-restricted diet without medical therapy), and type 2 diabetes mellitus (diet controlled without medical therapy).

An electrocardiogram, obtained within 10 minutes of arrival at the emergency department, showed ST elevation of 3 to 4 mm anteriorly. On coronary angiography, performed within 58 minutes of presentation, a completely occluded proximal left anterior descending (LAD) artery and 40%, 50%, and 50% stenoses of the proximal, middle, and distal portions of the right coronary artery (RCA), respectively, were noted. A left ventriculogram revealed akinesia of the anterior wall, anterior septum, and left ventricular (LV) apex, with an estimated LV ejection fraction (LVEF) of 25%.

MT underwent primary percutaneous coronary intervention (PCI) with implantation of a second-generation drug-eluting stent, which successfully restored patency of the LAD artery. On day 2 after PCI, he seemed to be doing relatively well, with no overt ischemic symptoms on ambulation. Occasional premature ventricular contractions (PVCs) were noted on telemetry, without evidence of sustained ventricular tachycardia (VT). His LVEF was 30% as determined by echocardiography.

1. In preparing MT for hospital discharge, which one of the following clinical findings would be an immediate concern?

A. Comorbid conditions.　　　　　　　B. LV dysfunction.

C. Stent thrombosis.　　　　　　　　D. Stenoses of the RCA.

2. Is MT a candidate for an implantable cardioverter-defibrillator (ICD) before hospital discharge for the primary prevention of SCD?

A. Yes, he is at high risk for SCD given his depressed LVEF.

B. No, he has no previous cardiac arrest.

C. Yes, his PVCs predispose him to SCD.

D. No, a waiting period is required before ICD consideration.

3. Medical Therapy.

Before discharge, appropriate pharmacotherapy was initiated and/or optimized in MT, including anti-platelet therapies (adenosine diphosphate receptor inhibitors and aspirin) for prevention of stent thrombosis and a β-blocker, an angiotensin-converting enzyme (ACE) inhibitor, and a statin (atorvastatin was optimized) for primary prevention of SCD.

What other therapy recommended for primary prevention of SCD should be added to MT's discharge medications?

A. Aldosterone antagonist.　　　　　　B. Amiodarone.

C. Atorvastatin.　　　　　　　　　　D. Hydralazine-nitrates.

4. Is MT a candidate for a WCD at hospital discharge?

A. No, he does not have a history of VA.

B. Yes, during the waiting period before ICD consideration.

C. No, he does not have a history of syncope.

D. Yes, indefinitely because he is at high risk.

5. Post-discharge follow-Up.

After discharge, MT was followed every month for the next 3 months. During this period, his medical therapies were further optimized and their adherence ascertained. At his 4-month-follow-up visit, a repeated echocardiogram revealed an LVEF of 42%.

Would you recommend an ICD for MT at this time?

A. Yes, he is still at high risk for SCD/SCA.

B. No, his LV function has improved.

C. Not before electrophysiologic evaluation.

D. Yes, but with cardiac resynchronization therapy capability as well.

Terminology related to cardiology department

congestive failure　充血性心脏衰竭

heart failure　心力衰竭

arrhythmia　心律失常

sinus tachycardia　窦性心动过速

sinus bradycardia　窦性心动过缓

sinus pause　窦性暂停

sinus arrest　窦性停搏

sinoatrial block　窦房传导阻滞

sick sinus syndrome　病态窦房结综合征

atrial premature beats　房性期前收缩

atrial tachycardia　房性心动过速

atrial flutter　心房扑动

atrial fibrillation　心房颤动

premature atrioventricular junctional beats　交界性期前收缩

atrioventricular junctional escape beats　房室交界性逸搏

nonparoxysmal atrioventricular junctional tachycardia　非阵发性房室交界性心动过速

paroxysmal supraventricular tachycardia　阵发性室上性心动过速

preexcitation syndrome　预激综合征

premature ventricular beats　室性期前收缩

ventricular tachycardia　室性心动过速

ventricular flutter　心室扑动

ventricular fibrillation　心室颤动

atrioventricular block　房室传导阻滞

intraventricular block　室内阻滞

right bundle branch block　右束支阻滞

left bundle branch block　左束支阻滞

left anterior fascicular block　左前分支阻滞

left posterior fascicular block　左后分支阻滞

sudden cardiac death　心脏性猝死

artificial cardiac pacing　人工心脏起搏

cardioversion　心脏电复律

congenital cardiovascular diseases　先天性心脏病

hypertension　高血压

primary hypertension　原发性高血压

secondary hypertension　继发性高血压

atherosclerosis　动脉粥样硬化

coronary atherosclerotic heart diseases　冠状动脉粥样硬化性心脏病

ischemic heart diseases　缺血性心脏病

angina pectoris 心绞痛

myocardial infarction 心肌梗死

rupture of the heart 心脏破裂

latent coronary heart diseases 无症状型冠心病

sudden death 猝死

mitral stenosis 二尖瓣狭窄

mitral incompetence 二尖瓣关闭不全

aortic stenosis 主动脉瓣狭窄

aortic incompetence 主动脉瓣关闭不全

tricuspid stenosis 三尖瓣狭窄

tricuspid incompetence 三尖瓣关闭不全

pulmonary stenosis 肺动脉狭窄

pulmonary incompetence 肺动脉瓣关闭不全

cardiomyopathy 心肌病

dilated cardiomyopathy 扩张型心肌病

hypertrophic cardiomyopathy 肥厚型心肌病

restrictive cardiomyopathy 限制型心肌病

pericardial diseases 心包疾病

syphilitic cardiovascular diseases 梅毒性心血管病

cardiovascular neurosis 心血管神经症

apical impulse 心尖搏动

thrill 震颤

palpable friction rubs (friction fremitus) 摩擦性震颤

heart rate 心率

cardiac rhythm 心律

sinus arrhythmia 窦性心律不齐

premature beat 期前收缩

pulse deficit 脉搏短绌

heart sound 心音

first heart sound 第一心音

second heart sound 第二心音

third heart sound 第三心音

fourth heart sound 第四心音

splitting of heart sound 心音分裂

extra cardiac sound 额外心音

gallop rhythm 奔马律

protodiastolic gallop 舒张早期奔马律

late diastolic gallop 舒张晚期奔马律

summation gallop 重叠性奔马律

opening snap 开瓣音

pericardial knock 心包叩击音

tumor plop 肿瘤扑落音

early systolic ejection sound 收缩早期喷射音

mid and late systolic click 收缩中晚期喀喇音

cardiac murmur 心脏杂音

systolic murmur 收缩期杂音

diastolic murmur 舒张期杂音

continuous murmurs 连续性杂音

crescendo murmur 递增型杂音

decrescendo murmur 递减型杂音

crescendo-decrescendo murmur 递增 - 递减型杂音

pericardial friction sound 心包摩擦音

pistol shot sound 枪击音

arteriosclerosis 动脉硬化症

hypertension 高血压病

acute myocarditis 急性心肌炎

valvular disease 心脏瓣膜病

infective endocarditis 感染性心内膜炎

electrocardiography（ECG/EKG）心电图

aberrant conduction 差异性传导

abnormal T wave T 波异常

absolute refractory period 绝对不应期

accelerated idioventricular rhythm 加速性室性自主心律

accelerated rhythm 加速性心律

advanced A-V block 重度房室传导阻滞

amplitude 幅度

anomalous atrioventricular conduction 异常房室传导

anterior myocardial infarction 前壁心肌梗死

antero-septal myocardial infarction 前间壁心肌梗死

antegrade conduction 顺向传导

anterolateral myocardial infarction 前侧壁心肌梗死

arrest 停搏

arrhythmia 心律失常

artifact 伪影

asystole 停搏

atrial arrhythmia 房性心律失常

atrial enlargement 心房扩大

atrial synchronous ventricular pacemaker 房室同步起搏器

atrioventricular block 房室传导阻滞

atrioventricular conduction ratio 房室传导比

atrioventricular dissociation 房室分离

atrioventricular junction 房室交界区

atrioventricular node 房室结

atropine test 阿托品试验

augmented lead 加压导联

AV sequential pacemaker 房室顺序起搏器

AVNRT/A-V node re-entry tachycardia 房室结折返性心动过速

AVRT/A-V re-entry tachycardia 房室折返性心动过速

Baseline 基线

bi-directional ventricular tachycardia 双向性室性心动过速

bifascicular block 双分支阻滞

bigeminy 二联律

bipolar lead 双极导联

blocked PAC 房性期前收缩未下传

bradycardia 心动过缓

Brugada syndrome 布鲁加综合征

bundle branch block 束支传导阻滞

capture 夺获

cardiac vector 心向量

coarse atrial fibrillation 粗房颤

compensatory pause 代偿间歇

concealed conduction 隐匿性传导

conduction system 传导系统

corrected QT interval 校正 QT 间期

coupling interval 配对间期

DDD pacemaker DDD 起搏器

decremental conduction 递减性传导

deflection 偏离

delta wave 预激波

double masters exercise test 二级梯运动试验

dual-chamber pacemaker 双腔起搏器

ectopic beat 异位搏动

electrical axis 电轴

electrical vector 电向量

end-diastolic PVC 舒张末期室性期前收缩

enhanced automaticity 自律性增高

escape rhythm 逸搏心律

exit block 传出阻滞

extensive anterior MI 广泛前壁心梗

F wave F 波

fascicular block 束支传导阻滞

fibrillation 颤动

atrial fibrillation 房颤

first degree 一度

flutter 扑动

full compensatory pause 代偿间期完全

fusion beat 融合波

high-degree atrioventricular block 高度房室传导阻滞

Holter 动态心电图

idionodal rhythm 结性自主心律

idioventricular 室性自主性

incomplete compensatory pause 代偿间歇不完全

inferior MI 下壁心肌梗死

interference and dissociation 干扰和脱节

interpolated PVC 间位性室性期前收缩

inverted T wave T 波倒置

irregular 不规则 / 不齐

junctional escape rhythm 交界性逸搏心律

lateral MI 侧壁心肌梗死

LBBB 左束支传导阻滞

lead 导联

left anterior fascicular block 左前分支阻滞

left axis deviation 电轴左偏

long Q-T syndrome 长 Q-T 综合征

loose electrode 电极松动

low voltage 低电压

Lown-Ganong-Levine syndrome L-G-L 综合征

LVH/left ventricular hypertrophy 左心室肥厚

marked bradycardia　显著心动过缓

MI/myocardial infarction　心肌梗死

monophasic curve　单向曲线

multifocal PVC　多源性室性期前收缩

multiform PVC　多形性室性期前收缩

multistage stress test　多级运动试验

myocardial ischemia　心肌缺血

Non-Q wave MI　非 Q 波性心梗

nonsustained ventricular tachycardia　非持续性室性心动过速

nontransmural MI　非透壁性心梗

normal sinus rhythm　正常窦性心律

P mitrale　二尖瓣型 P 波

P Pulmonale　肺型 P 波

PAC/premature atrial contractions　房性期前收缩

pacemaker rhythm　起搏心律

paired PVC　成对室性期前收缩

para-systole　并行心律

paroxysmal junctional (supraventricular)tachycardia　阵发性交界 (室上) 性心动过速

peri-infarction block　梗死周围阻滞

posterior MI　后壁心梗

P-P interval　P-P 间期

P-R interval　P-R 间期

P-R segment　P-R 段

pre-cordial leads　胸前导联

pre-excitation syndrome　预激综合征

pulseless electrical activity　无脉性电活动

PVC/premature ventricular contractions　室性期前收缩

Q (q) wave　Q(q) 波

QRS Complex　QRS 波

Q-T interval　Q-T 间期

Quadrigeminy　四联律

RBBB　右束支传导阻滞

reciprocal rhythm　反复心律

right axis deviation　电轴右偏

R-on-T phenomenon　R-on-T 现象

R-R interval　R-R 间期

RVH/Right Ventricular Hypertrophy　右室肥厚

second degree 二度

secondary changes 继发性改变

septal MI 间隔心梗

sick sinus syndrome(SSS) 病态窦房结综合征

sinoatrial block 窦房传导阻滞

sinus arrest 窦性停搏

sinus arrhythmia 窦性心律不齐

sinus bradycardia 窦性心动过缓

sinus P wave 窦性 P 波

sinus tachycardia 窦性心动过速

speed of ECG paper 心电图纸走速

ST segment depression ST 段压低

standard limb leads 标准肢体导联

standstill 静止

strain 劳损

subepicardial ischemia 心外膜下缺血

supraventricular 室上性

T wave T 波

Ta wave 心房复极波

Tachycardia 心动过速

TDP/torsade de pointes 尖端扭转型室性心动过速

third degree 三度

TP segment TP 段

treadmill test 运动平板试验

trifascicular block 三分支阻滞

trigemini 三联律

U wave U 波

unifocal PVC 单源室性期前收缩

VAT/ventricular activation time 心室激动时间

ventricular enlargement 心室扩大

ventricular fibrillation 室性颤动

ventricular flutter 室性扑动

VT/ventricular tachycardia 室性心动过速

Chapter 3

Respiratory System

Section A　Focus Listening

Conversation

Listen to the dialogue and fill in the blanks with proper words.

D=doctor　P=patient

D: Hello, take a seat, would you please tell me what the problem is?

P: Thank you, Doctor, I've come to see you because I had a cough, but I also seem to wheeze a lot, and it is not getting any better.

D: Is this a recent _____, or have you had it for some time?

P: For some time, Doctor.

D: Do you suffer from coughing fits (cough a lot)?

P: Yes, a lot.

D: Do you cough up phlegm or is it a dry cough?

P: I _____ quite a bit of phlegm. I'm afraid I have asthma. Tens should be taken into consideration.

D: What is the phlegm like?

P: What do you mean?

D: Can you describe the phlegm for me? What color is it? Yellow or greenish, and is it _____ or sticky?

P: Yes, it's yellowish and kind of looks like jelly.

D: Does it have a smell?

P: No, I don't think so.

D: Has there ever been _____ in it?

P: Yes, just once I some blood in it.

D: Have you taken any medicine or _____ recently?

P: Yes, I was on something to thin my blood.

New Words & Expressions

cough fit 咳嗽一阵子   bring up 呕吐

frothy 泡沫的；泡沫般的   jelly 胶冻；胶状物

tablet 药片

Passage

Answer the questions after listening to the passage.

1. Which part of the lung is damaged in Emphysema?

A. Alveoli.   B. Bronchi.   C. Bronchioles.   D. All of the above.

2. Which one of the following terms refers to the worsening of symptoms in COPD?

A. Extrusion.   B. Extraction.   C. Exacerbation.   D. Extension.

3. What is the meaning of the term sputum?

A. Excess production of blood.   B. Excess production of mucus in the lungs.

C. Excessive cough.   D. Excess water in the body.

4. What are the common risk factors for COPD?

A. Unhealthy air quality.   B. Smoking.

C. Alcohol consumption.   D. Both A and B.

5. Which one of the following is the characteristic feature of COPD?

A. More inflated lungs.   B. Less inflated lungs.

C. No inflation of lungs.   D. None of the above.

Section B   Reading Comprehension

Text

A 73-year-old woman presents to the emergency department (ED) with fever, chills, and night sweats. Approximately 3 weeks ago, the patient was hospitalized for hematochezia and fever. Urine cultures from that hospitalization had grown Escherichia coli, and the blood cultures were positive for Serratia marcescens. The workup during that initial hospitalization also included a transthoracic echocardiogram that revealed no valvular abnormalities, a non-contrast abdominal computed tomography (CT) scan, which failed to demonstrate any intra-abdominal pathology, and a colonoscopy, which was only positive for polyps. At the time of discharge, the hematochezia was suspected to have been caused by several large external hemorrhoids that were noted on the physical examination as a diagnosis of exclusion. A set of repeat blood cultures was performed, and they were negative for growth. The patient was discharged home to complete a 2-week course of levofloxacin after confirming sensitivities from the initial set of cultures.

At today's presentation to the ED (3 days after finishing her course of levofloxacin), the patient states that over the past 24 hours, the fever and chills have returned. She denies any rectal bleeding, dizziness, headache, chest pain, hematemesis, abdominal pain, melena, dysuria, or recent weight change. Her past medical history includes hypertension, abdominal aortic aneurysm with bilateral iliac artery occlusive disease, treated by aortobifemoral bypass grafting 6 years ago, coronary artery disease, treated with a coronary artery bypass grafting performed 1 year ago, diabetes; chronic renal insufficiency, and diverticulosis. She has an 80-pack-year history of smoking, and she currently continues to smoke. The review of systems is only notable for a chronic cough.

The physical examination demonstrates a toxic-appearing elderly woman who is actively experiencing rigors, with a temperature of 103.0℉ (39.4℃) and a heart rate of 104 bpm. Her blood pressure is stable at 120/86 mm Hg. She has a pulse oxygenation of 97% while breathing room air. There are distant and regular heart sounds, but no murmur is noted. The lung examination is unremarkable except for an occasional wheeze. The abdomen is soft and non-tender, with positive normoactive bowel sounds and no apparent organomegaly. She has a well-healed midline abdominal incision from her prior surgery. The rectal examination reveals several non-tender external hemorrhoids, with no evidence of recent bleeding. Guaiac testing of the stool is strongly positive.

Her laboratory findings are notable for a white blood cell (WBC) count of $23.7 \times 10^3/\mu L$ ($23.7 \times 10^9/L$), with 98% neutrophils and 12% bands; a hemoglobin of 8.2 g/dL (82 g/L) and a hematocrit of 24.6% (0.246; baseline hemoglobin was 10 g/dL and baseline hematocrit was 29.4% at time of discharge approximately 2 weeks ago), and a creatinine of 1.8 mg/dL (159.12 μmol/L). The liver transaminases are within normal limits. A urinalysis is unremarkable. A chest x-ray shows clear lung fields. Given her relatively recent history of colonic instrumentation, a repeat abdominal CT scan is performed, this time with both oral and intravenous contrasts (see Figure 2).

To help making the diagnosis, additional information from the hospitalization is presented here. Two sets of

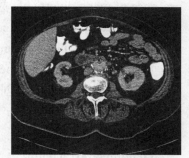

Figure 2　Image of abdominal CT scan

blood cultures were drawn in the ED, at the time of initial presentation, several hours apart, and the 2 cultures were noted to be positive for different organisms: Alpha-hemolytic Streptococcus and Candida glabrata. Additionally, a repeat echocardiogram was again negative for vegetations.

New Words & Expressions

culture ['kʌltʃə] *v.* to grow bacteria or cells for medical or scientific use 培养 [细菌或细胞]

escherichia coli [ˌɛʃəˈrɪkɪə] *n.* [细菌] 大肠埃希杆菌，大肠杆菌 [亦称作 Ecoli]

serratia marcescens 灵杆菌；黏质沙雷菌

transthoracic [ˌtrænsθəˈræsɪk] *a.* done or made by way of the thoracic cavity 经胸廓的，经胸腔的

echocardiogram[ˌekəʊˈkɑ:dɪəgræm] *n.* a visual record made by echocardiography; also the procedure for producing such a record 超声心动图

workup ['wɜ:kʌp] *n.* an intensive diagnostic study 诊断检查

colonoscope [kəˈlɒnəskəʊp] *n.* endoscopic examination of the colon 结肠镜

polyp ['pɒlɪp] *n.* a growth projecting from a mucous membrane 息肉

hemorrhoid [ˌheməˈrɔɪd] *n.* 痔疮

levofloxacin [levəflɒkˈseɪsɪn] *n.* 左氧氟沙星

hematemesis [ˌhiməˈteməsɪs] *n.* bright red blood is vomited, often associated with esophageal varices or peptic ulcer 呕血，吐血

dysuria [dɪsˈjʊərɪə] *n.* difficult or painful discharge of urine 排尿困难

aneurysm ['ænjərɪzəm] *n.* an abnormal blood-filled bulge of a blood vessel and especially an artery resulting from weakening (as from disease) of the vessel wall 动脉瘤

iliac ['ɪlɪæk] *n.* of, relating to, or located near the ilium 髂骨的

occlusive [əˈklu:sɪv] *a.* characterized by occlusion 闭塞的；有闭塞倾向的

aortobifemoral [eɪɔ:təʊbɪˈfemərəl] *a.* 主动脉与两侧股动脉的

diverticulosis [ˌdaɪvəˌtɪkjəˈləʊsɪs] *n.* an intestinal disorder characterized by the presence of many diverticula 憩室病

rigor ['rɪgə] *n.* a tremor caused by a chill 发烧前的寒战

oxygenation [ˌɒksɪdʒəˈneɪʃ(ə)n] *n.* 以氧处理；氧化作用

organomegaly ['ɔ:gənɒmegəlɪ] *n.* the abnormal enlargement of organs 器官巨大症

guaiac ['gwaɪæk] *n.* 愈创木脂

neutrophil ['nju:trəfil] *n.* a granulocyte that is the chief phagocytic white blood cell of the blood 中性粒细胞

creatinine [kriˈætənin] *n.* 肌酸酐

transaminase [trænsˈæməˌneɪs] *n.* an enzyme promoting transamination (aminotransferase)

转氨酶

urinalysis [jʊrə'næləsɪs] *n.* chemical analysis of urine 尿分析

Exercise

Decide whether the following statements are true (T) or false (F) according to the passage.

_____1. The workup during that initial hospitalization also included a transthoracic echocardiogram that revealed valvular abnormalities.

_____2. The patient's past medical history includes hypertension; abdominal aortic aneurysm with bilateral iliac artery occlusive disease, treated by aortobifemoral bypass grafting 6 years ago.

_____3. The abdomen is soft and non-tender, with negative normoactive bowel sounds and no apparent organomegaly.

_____4. Given her relatively recent history of colonic instrumentation, a repeat abdominal CT scan is performed, this time with both oral and intravenous contrasts.

_____5. She has a pulse oxygenation of 98% while breathing room air.

Answer the following questions according to the passage.

1. What is the most likely origin of these recurrent bloodstream infections?

_____

2. What was the patient hospitalized for approximately 3 weeks ago?

_____

3. What therapeutic schedule can you provide?

_____

Use the appropriate form of the words or phrases in the box to complete the following sentences.

echocardiogram	hematemesis	dysuria	incision	colonoscopy
diverticulosis	hematochezia	urinalysis	wheeze	aneurysm
dizziness	organisms	culture		

1._____was the main syndrome of rectal cancer and it happened more commonly in old age than younger cases, but the abdominal pain was lowered than that in younger ones.

2. It's a common medical sense that _____ is a procedure enabling your surgeon to examine the lining of the rectum and colon.

3. A 40-year-old male presented with severe _____ and shock status after several days of abdominal discomfort.

4. The doctor listened to her heart, which had a normal rhythm, and to her lungs, hearing the fine crackles of pulmonary fibrosis but also a new_____.

5. A traditional, open procedure using a larger _____ may be required to safely remove the infected appendix in these patients.

6. Sugar can be measured in the urine through a lab test commonly called a _____ _____.

7. Bacteria are among the simplest _____ in nature, but many of them can still talk to each other, using a chemical "language" that is critical to the process of infection.

8. _____ provides information about the size and shape of your heart and how well your heart chambers and valves are functioning.

9. It may help in the prevention of colon cancer and it is helpful in preventing _____ _____ and hemorrhoids.

10. This causes a range of problems from headaches, nausea, and _____ to cardiovascular problems and confusion.

Translation

A. Translate the following expressions into English.

1. 肝转氨酶
2. 无痛性外痔
3. 大肠杆菌
4. 愈创木脂法粪便检测
5. 冠状动脉旁路移植术
6. 慢性肾功能不全
7. 尿液培养
8. 排除诊断

B. Translate the following sentences or expressions into Chinese.

1. To help in making the diagnosis, additional information from the hospitalization is presented here.

2. The patient was discharged to home to complete a 2-week course of levofloxacin after confirming sensitivities from the initial set of cultures.

3. The physical examination demonstrates a toxic-appearing elderly woman who is actively experiencing rigors, with a temperature of 103.0℉ (39.4℃) and a heart rate of 104 bpm.

4. At the time of discharge, the hematochezia was suspected to have been caused by several large external hemorrhoids.

5. At today's presentation to the ED (3 days after her course of levofloxacin), the patient states that over the past 24 hours，the fever and chills have returned.

Section C   Vocabulary (Terminology)

1. 呼吸 breath

Combining Form	Meaning	Terminology	Terminology meaning
spiro-	breathing	spirometer	an instrument for measuring the air entering and leaving the lungs 呼吸量计；肺活（量）计
pneumato-	1. respiration 2. air, vapor, gas	pneumatosis	积气症（少用）
-pnea	breathing	tachypnea	excessively rapid and shallow breathing, hyperventilation 呼吸急促
pneumo pneumono-	air, lung,	pneumothorax	a condition in which air or other gas is present in the pleural cavity and which occurs spontaneously as a result of disease or injury of lung tissue, rupture of air-filled pulmonary cysts, or puncture of the chest wall or is induced as a therapeutic measure to collapse the lung 气胸

2. 鼻 nose

Combining Form	Meaning	Terminology	Terminology meaning
naso-	nose	nasogastric intubation	being or performed by intubation of the stomach through the nasal passage 鼻胃插管法
rhino-	nose	rhinoplasty	plastic surgery on the nose usually for cosmetic purposes 鼻整形术

3. 喉 throat

Combining Form	Meaning	Terminology	Terminology meaning
laryngo-	larynx, voice box	laryngospasm	spasmodic closure of the larynx 喉痉挛

4. 咽 pharynx

Combining Form	Meaning	Terminology	Terminology meaning
pharyngo-	pharynx, throat	pharyngeal	relating to or located or produced in the region of the pharynx 咽的

5. 声门 glottis

Combining Form	Meaning	Terminology	Terminology meaning
glotto-		glottiscope	声门镜

6. 气管 trachea, windpipe

Combining Form	Meaning	Terminology	Terminology meaning
tracheo-	trachea, windpipe	tracheotomy	the surgical operation of cutting into the trachea especially through the skin 气管切开术

7. 支气管 bronchus

Combining Form	Meaning	Terminology	Terminology meaning
broncho-	bronchus, bronchial tube	bronchodilator	a drug that relaxes bronchial muscle resulting in expansion of the bronchial air passages 支气管扩张剂
bronchio-	bronchus, bronchial tube	bronchiectasis	a chronic dilatation of bronchi or bronchioles 支气管扩张
bronchiolo-	bronchiole, small bronchus	bronchiolitis	inflammation of the bronchioles 细支气管炎

8. 肺 lung

Combining Form	Meaning	Terminology	Terminology meaning
pulmono-	lung	pulmonary	of, relating to, affecting, or occurring in the lungs 肺的；肺病的
pneumono-		pneumonectomy	excision of an entire lung or of one or more lobes of a lung 肺切除

9. 肺泡 alveolus, air sacs

Combining Form	Meaning	Terminology	Terminology meaning
alveolo-	alveolus, air sac	alveolar	of, relating to, resembling, or having alveoli 肺泡的；小泡状的

10. 胸膜 pleura

Combining Form	Meaning	Terminology	Terminology meaning
pleuro-	pleura	pleurodynia	pain in the chest wall that is aggravated by breathing 胸膜痛

11.epiglottis 会厌

Combining Form	Meaning	Terminology	Terminology meaning
epiglotto-	epiglottis	epiglottitis	inflammation of epiglottis which are characterized by fever, sore throat, and an erythematous, swollen epiglottis 会厌炎

12. 扁桃体 tonsil

Combining Form	Meaning	Terminology	Terminology meaning
tonsillo-	tonsils	tonsillectomy	the oropharyngeal tonsils are removed 扁桃体切除术

13. 呼吸系统常用的前缀、后缀：

Combining Form	Meaning	Terminology	Terminology meaning
ortho-	straight, upright	orthopnea	an abnormal condition in which breathing is easier in the upright position 端坐呼吸
oxo-	oxygen	hypoxia	deficiency of oxygen reaching the tissues of the body 组织缺氧

续表

Combining Form	Meaning	Terminology	Terminology meaning
phono-	voice	dysphonia	defective use of the voice 发声困难；言语障碍
phreno	diaphragm	phrenic nerve	the motor nerve to the diaphragm 膈神经
sinuso-	sinus, cavity	sinusitis	inflammation of a sinus 窦炎
-ema	condition	empyema	the presence of pus in a bodily cavity 积脓
-osmia	smell	anosmia	loss or impairment of the sense of smell 嗅觉丧失症
-ptysis	spitting	hemoptysis	expectoration of blood from some part of the respiratory tract 咳血
-sphyxia	pulse	asphyxia	lack of pulse due to lack of oxygen 无脉症
-thorax	pleural cavity, chest	pyothorax	empyema of the chest 脓胸

Exercise for vocabulary

Select the proper meaning from column II to match column I.

	I		II
(	) 1. bronho-	A.	voice box
(	) 2. laryngo-	B.	chest
(	) 3. alveolo-	C.	straight, upright
(	) 4. bronchiolo-	D.	pleura
(	) 5. ortho-	E.	breathing
(	) 6. pleuro- larynx	F.	smell
(	) 7. pneumo-	G.	bronchus, bronchial tube
(	) 8. spiro-	H.	air, lung
(	) 9. thoraco-	I.	small bronchus
(	) 10. -osma	J.	air sac

	I		II
(	) 1. -sphyxia	A.	condition
(	) 2. tracheo-	B.	breathing
(	) 3. -ema	C.	nose
(	) 4. -pnea	D.	pleural cavity, chest
(	) 5. naso-	E.	tonsils
(	) 6. -thorax	F.	spitting
(	) 7. tonsillo-	G.	throat
(	) 8. -ptysis	H.	wind pip
(	) 9. pharyngo-	I.	voice
(	) 10. phono-	J.	pulse

Match the following pathological conditions or terms with their meanings below.

orthopnea	empyema	hemoptysis	pyothorax	tonsillectomy
pleurodynia	pneumonectomy	bronchiolitis	bronchiectasisalveolar	
bronchodilator	tracheotomy	laryngospasm	nasogastric intubation	
pneumothorax	tachypnea	spirometer		

_____1. Being performed by intubation of the stomach through the nasal passage.

_____2. A drug that relaxes bronchial muscle resulting in expansion of the bronchial air passages.

_____3. Expectoration of blood from some parts of the respiratory tract.

_____4. The oropharyngeal tonsils are removed.

_____5. Spasmodic closure of the larynx.

_____6. Excision of an entire lung or of one or more lobes of a lung.

_____7. The surgical operation of cutting into the trachea especially through the skin.

_____8. Excessively rapid and shallow breathing, hyperventilation.

_____9. A condition in which air or other gas is present in the pleural cavity and which occurs spontaneously, as a result of disease or injury to lung tissue. Rupture of air-filled pulmonary cysts, or puncture of the chest wall or is induced as a therapeutic measure to collapse the lung.

_____10. A chronic dilatation of bronchi or bronchioles.

_____11. Pain in the chest wall that is aggravated by breathing.

_____12. The presence of pus in a bodily cavity.

_____13. Of, relating to, resembling, or having alveoli.

_____14. An instrument for measuring the air entering and leaving the lungs.

_____15. Inflammation of the bronchioles.

_____16. Empyema of the chest.

_____17. An abnormal condition in which breathing is easier in the upright position.

Choose the term that best completes the meaning of the sentence.

1. A 16-year-old female produced yellow-colored sputum and had a high fever, the physician told her that she probably had_____ and needed antibiotics.

    A. pneumonia.   B. pulmonary embolism.

    C. pneumothorax.   D. lung cancer.

2. Dr. Wang used his stethoscope to perform _____ on the patient chest.

    A. percussion.   B. auscultation.

C. thoracentesis.   D. inspection.

3. Mr. Xu, 76-year-old, had been a pack-a-day smoker all his life. Over the previous 3 months he noticed a persistent cough, weight loss, blood in her sputum _____and dyspnea, A chest CT revealed a mass. Biopsy confirmed the diagnosis of _____, which is a type of_____ lung cancer.

A. hemoptysis, adenocarcinoma, non-small cell.

B. hematemesis, tuberculosis, small cell.

C. asbestosis, pneumoconiosis lymph node.

D. hemoptysis, adenocarcinoma, small cell.

4. An aged male presented with history of chronic productive cough for over 20 years, and tachypnea and asthma for 6 ~ 7years also complaining of aggravated cough productive of purulent sputum for past 10 days. On examination: diminished breathing sound, scattered wheezing heard, moist rales heard in both middle and lower lung field. FEV1/FVC ratio: 50%, the total lung capacity (TLC) account for 68% the expected total lung capacity, blood picture: WBC 1.8×10^9/L, N 0.82. What's the best diagnosis?

A. Chronic bronchitis, COPD (chronic obstructive pulmonary disease).

B. Chronic bronchitis with pulmonary infection, COPD.

C. Bronchial asthma with pulmonary infection, COPD.

D. Bronchiectasis with pulmonary infection, COPD.

5. A middle aged male complained of recurrent cough productive of purulent sputum for many years. On examination: obesity, breathing sound symmetrically heard on both lungs. Much moist rales heard on both lungs. The pulmonary function test showed: FEV1 60%, $PaCO_2$ 65mmHg, PaO_2 56mmHg, hematocrit 65%, chest fluoroscopy showed: both lung markings increased and intensification of lung markings, the heart shadow slightly enlarged. The patient should be diagnosed with _____.

A. chronic lung abscess.

B. bronchiectasis with infection.

C. obstructive pulmonary emphysema (pink puffer).

D. obstructive pulmonary emphysema (blue bloater).

6. A 40-year-old male complained of cold intolerance, fever and headache due to getting wet 5 or 6 days ago, however, chest tightness and tachypnea presented from this morning. On examination: orthopnea, slightly cyanosis over the lips, barrel chest, wheezing heard over both lungs, the routine blood test is in normal limits. The patient stated he had similar attack before this attack. So, what's the most likely diagnosis?

A. Influenza.   B. Bronchial asthma.

C. Lobar pneumonia.   D. Cardiac asthma.

7. A 45-year-old male with history of tuberculosis and recurrent episode of asthma

complained of sudden onset of dyspnea and right chest pain half an hour ago when walking up stairs. On examination: obvious dyspnea, cyanosis, orthopnea, drenching sweats, vexation, engorgement of jugular veins, slightly leftward of trachea, barrel chest, lungs present hyperresonance on percussion, the light lung presents slight tympany except hyperresonance, diminished breathing sound heard in right lung, the wheezing heard in left lung. What's the probable diagnosis?

A. Acute episode bronchial asthma.

B. Tuberculosis with bronchial asthma.

C. Bronchial asthma with spontaneous pneumothorax.

D. Asthma with pleural effusion.

8. Mr. Liu, aged 56, complained of fever and cough a month ago, he stated that he has history of fever, cough productive of trace white and stick sputum 7 months ago, the chest fluoroscopy showed a patchy density over the upper right lung. He also stated the similar episode presented 5 months ago. On examination: diminished breathing sound in the upper right lung without rales, blood picture showed: WBC 11.5×10^9/L, N 0.82, L 0.18 chest fluoroscopy showed a big patchy high density over the upper right lung. What would the most likely diagnosis be?

A. Mycoplasma pneumonia.   B. Viral pneumonia.

C. Obstructive pneumonia.   D. Tuberculosis.

9. A 45-year-old male complained of tachypnea and dry cough for 3 years. He denied a history of arthropathy. On examination: normal temperature and blood pressure, pulse 90 beats/min, respiration 30/min, slightly cyanosed lips, acropachy, moist rales heard in both lungs, Chest fluoroscopy showed small density nodule. The lab findings show RF positive, LDH 600U, pulmonary function tests showed restrictive ventilation disorder. What's the diagnosis?

A. Chronic bronchitis.   B. Idiopathic pulmonary fibrosis.

C. Metastatic lung cancer.   D. Bronchiectasis with lung infections.

10. A 60-year-old male with history of recurrent productive cough for 20 years complained of aggravated tachypnea and cough productive of purulent sputum for a week. He stated the tachypnea after exercise presented in past 7 to 8 years. On examination: heart rate 130 bpm, blowing systolic murmur heard in tricuspid region, emphysema sign found in both lungs, moist rales and wheezes heard in both lungs, the liver palpable 3 cm below the coastal margin with soft consistency and tenderness. Hepatojugular reflux positive, edema found in both lower limbs, ECG shows RV1+SV5=1.3mV. Chest fluoroscopy shows 18mm of transverse diameter of pulmonary artery stem in lower right lung. What's the most likely diagnosis?

A. Chronic bronchitis, pulmonary emphysema, lung infection.

B. Respiratory failure due to pulmonary emphysema.

C. Chronic pulmonary heart disease with coronary heart disease.

D. Acute exacerbating phase of chronic pulmonary heart disease.

Section D   Writing

在上章节里我们大概地了解了英文病历的原貌，我们现在正式开始写英文病历，一个完整的英文住院病历分为 13 个部分，即：

1. 一般项目 (General data)；

2. 主诉 (CC)；

3. 现病史 (HPI)；

4. 既往史 (PMH)；

5. 药物史 (Med)；

6. 过敏史 (All)；

7. 家庭史 (FHx)；

8. 社会史 (SHx)；

9. 系统回顾 (ROS)；

10. 体格检查 (PE)；

11. 实验室及数据资料 (Lab/Data)；

12. 病史小结 / 初步诊断 / 病历摘要；

13. 诊疗计划。

我们就英文病历写作各个部分逐一讲解，确定和解释各部分的目的并举例说明。首先，我们来谈谈一般项目的写作。一般项目包括姓名 (name)、年龄 (age)、性别 (sex)、职业 (occupation)、住址 (有的会包括临时住址以及永久住址)(address)、婚姻状况 (marital state)、种族 (race)、国籍 (nationality)、住院时间 (date of admission)、病史采集时间 (date history taken)。

Patient's Name

Insist on recording the complete name, including the family name and all given names. The family name should be placed first, followed by a comma and all given names. Be careful to obtain the correct spelling. Any file of considerable size contains the records of several patients.

例：

Name: Mathew M Hilton

Age: 37 years old

Sex: male

Occupation: retired staff

Address: 56, Yangming Road, Donghu district, Nanchang, Jiangxi.

Marital Status: married

Race: Han

Nationality: China

Date of Admission: Aug.16th, 2017

Date history taken: 11:15 AM, Aug.16th, 2017

我们国家的病历与英美国家的相比更复杂一些，比如在一般项目里多了籍贯、身份证号码、工作单位及电话、联系人电话、病史陈述者、病史可靠程度等。

Name:

Age:

Sex:

Occupation:

Date of birth:

Marital status:

Race:

Place of birth (birth place):

Nationality:

Code of ID card:

Work place and TEL:

Address and TEL:

Person to notify and TEL:

Source of history:

Reliability of history:

Date of admission:

Date history taken:

在英文病历中如何写好这部分，我们在此详细阐述。

1. 年龄的表示方法（以 28 岁为例）

28 years old (y/o)

age 28

28-year-old

the age of 28

28 years of age

2. 性别的表示方法

male, ♂ 男性

female, ♀ 女性

3. 职业的表示方法

工人：worker

退休工人：retired worker

农民：farmer (peasant)

干部：leader (cadre)

行政人员：administrative personnel (staff)

职员：staff member

商人：trader (businessman)

教师：teacher

学生：student

医生：doctor

药剂师：pharmacist

护士：nurse

军人：soldier

警察：policeman

工程师：engineer

技术员：technician

家政人员：housekeeper

家庭主妇：housewife

营业员：assistant

服务员：attendant

售票员：conductor

4. 民族的表示方法

汉：Han

回：Hui

蒙：Meng

藏：Tibetan

朝鲜：Korean

5. 日期的表示方法

2007 年 10 月 1 日 [10-1-2007(10/1/2007; Oct.1,2007; Oct.1st,2007)](美国)

2007 年 10 月 1 日 [1-10-2007(1/10/2007; 1 Oct.,2007; 1st of Oct.,2007)] (英国)

6. 婚姻状况的表示方法

已婚：married

未婚：single (unmarried)

离婚：divorced

寡妇：widow

鳏夫：widower

7. 病史可靠程度的表示方法

可靠：reliable

不可靠：unreliable

不完全可靠：not entirely

无法获得：unobtainable

8. 住址的表示方法：与英文住址的表达方法是一致的，以从小至大的顺序排列。

如：江西省南昌市阳明路 56 号

NO.56, Yangming Road, Nanchang, Jiangxi

江西省莲花县坪里乡五洲村

Wuzhou Village, Pingli Township, Lianhua County, Jiangxi

9. 病史陈述者的表示方法

患者本人：Patient himself (herself)

患者的丈夫：Her husband

患者的妻子：His wife

患者的同事：Patient's colleague

患者的邻居：Patient's neighbor

患者的亲属 (父亲、母亲、儿子、女儿、兄弟、姐妹)：Patient's kin (father, mother, son, daughter, brother, sister),

Exercise

Write the general items in a medical record according to the following content.

贾某，女，56 岁，汉族，已婚，江西省南昌市人，会计师，家住南昌市西湖区，因突发性右侧肢体瘫痪于 2008 年 3 月 16 日入院。病史采集时间：2008 年 3 月 16 日 10：00AM，病情陈述由患者本人陈述，正确可靠。

Section E　Spoken English

Role play

Directions: A girl visited a doctor accompanied by her mother, the young girl had fever. 3 students work in pairs to demonstrate the conversation, one plays the role of doctor, the others of patient and mother respectively.

Discussion

Directions: Work in groups and discuss with your partners, then answer the following questions with detailed analysis.

A 64-year-old man with a history of chronic obstructive pulmonary disease (COPD) is evaluated in the emergency department for increased dyspnea over the past 48 hours. There is no change in his baseline production of white sputum but he has increased nasal congestion and sore throat. His medications include inhaled tiotropium, combination fluticasone and salmeterol, and albuterol.

The patient is alert but in mild respiratory distress. The temperature is 38.6℃ (101.5℉), blood pressure is 150/90 mmHg, pulse rate is 108/min, and respiration rate is 30/min. Oxygen saturation with the patient breathing ambient air is 90%. Breath sounds are diffusely decreased with bilateral expiratory wheezes; he is using accessory muscles to breathe. He does not have any peripheral edema or elevated jugular venous distension (JVD). With the patient breathing oxygen, 2 L/min by nasal cannula, arterial blood gases (ABGS) are PH 7.27, PCO_2 60 mmHg, and PO_2, 62 mmHg: oxygen saturation is 91%. His CBC shows leukocytosis of 11, 000 and chest x-ray does not show any new infiltrates or pneumothorax.

1. What is your diagnosis?
2. How would you approach this patient?

Terminology related to respiratory department

lobar pneumonia 大叶性肺炎
emphysema 肺气肿
hemoptysis 咯血
gasp 气喘
gas pain 气痛
lobular pneumonia 小叶性肺炎
bronchogenic carcinoma 支气管癌
pulmonary atelectasis 肺扩张不全
stridor 喘鸣
acute upper respiratory tract infection 急性上呼吸道感染
common cold 普通感冒
chronic bronchitis 慢性支气管炎
obstructive pulmonary emphysema 阻塞性肺气肿
cor pulmonale 肺源性心脏病
chronic pulmonary heart disease 慢性肺源性心脏病
acute cor pulmonale 急性肺源性心脏病
bronchial asthma 支气管哮喘
bronchiectasis 支气管扩张
bronchial asthma 支气管哮喘

respiratory failure　呼吸衰竭

acute respiratory distress syndrome　急性呼吸窘迫综合征

pneumonia　肺炎

pneumococcal pneumonia　肺炎球菌肺炎

staphylococcus pneumonia　葡萄球菌肺炎

klebsiella pneumonia　克雷白杆菌肺炎

legionnaires disease　军团病

mycoplasma pneumonia　支原体肺炎

pulmonary aspergillosis　肺曲菌病

lung abscess　肺脓肿

pulmonary tuberculosis　肺结核

interstitial lung disease　间质性肺疾病

idiopathic pulmonary fibrosis　特发性肺纤维化

pulmonary alveolar proteinosis　肺泡蛋白质沉积症

silicosis　矽肺

sarcoidosis　结节病

primary bronchogenic carcinoma　原发性支气管肺癌

lung cancer　肺癌

pneumothorax　气胸

spontaneous pneumothorax　自发性气胸

empyema　脓胸

pleuritis　胸膜炎

vocal fremitus　语音震颤

three depression sign　三凹征

dyspnea　呼吸困难

orthopnea　端坐呼吸

trepopnea　转卧呼吸

platypnea　平卧呼吸

tachypnea　呼吸急促

bradypnea　呼吸过缓

thoracic expansion　胸廓扩张度

pleural friction fremitus　胸膜摩擦感

indirect percussion　间接叩诊

direct percussion　直接叩诊

hyperresonance　过清音

amphorophony　空瓮音

breath sound　呼吸音

tracheal breath sound 气管呼吸音

bronchial breath sound 支气管音

bronchovesicular breath sound 支气管肺泡呼吸音

vesicular breath sound 肺泡呼吸音

rales 啰音

crackles 啰音

moist crackles 湿啰音

bubble sound 水泡音

coarse crackles 粗湿啰音

medium crackles 中湿啰音

fine crackles 细湿啰音

crepitus 捻发音

wheezes 干啰音

rhonchi 干啰音

sibilant wheezes 高调干啰音

sonorous wheezes 低调干啰音

vocal resonance 语音共振

bronchophony 支气管语音

pectoriloquy 胸语音

egophony 羊鸣音

pleural friction rub 胸膜摩擦音

pleural effusion 胸腔积液

basal lung volume 基础肺容积

basal lung capacity 基础肺容量

tidal volume 潮气容积

expiratory reserve volume 补呼气容积

inspiratory reserve volume 补吸气容积

inspiratory capacity 深吸气量

vital capacity 肺活量

functional residual capacity 功能残气量

residual capacity 残气量

minute ventilation 每分钟静息通气量

maximal voluntary ventilation 最大自主通气量

forced vital capacity 用力肺活量

maximal mid-expiratory flow 最大呼气中段流量

alveolar ventilation radius 肺泡通气量

peak expiratory flow 最大呼气量

gas distribution　气体分布

ventilation/perfusion ratio　通气 / 血流比值

alveolar diffusion capacity　肺弥散量

small airway function　小气道功能

regional lung function　区域性肺功能

closing volume　闭合容积

maximum expiratory flow-volume curve　最大呼气流量 - 容积曲线

blood gas analysis　血气分析

blood pH　血 pH

partial pressure of carbon dioxide(PCO_2)　二氧化碳分压

carbon dioxide combining power(CO_2CP)　二氧化碳结合力

standard bicarbonate(SB)　标准碳酸氢盐

actual bicarbonate(AB)　实际碳酸氢盐

buffer base(BB)　缓冲碱

base excess(BE)　剩余碱

total carbon dioxide(T CO_2)　二氧化碳总量

oxygen content(O_2-C)　氧含量

partial pressure of oxygen(PO_2)　氧分压

oxygen saturation(O_2sat or SaO_2)　血氧饱和度

Chapter 4

Digestive System

Section A   Focus Listening

Conversation

Listen to the dialogue and fill in the blanks with proper words.

D=doctor P=patient

D: Hello, I am Doctor Jiang. May I have your name and age?

P: My name is Wang Ning. I am 48 years old.

D: Mr. Wang. Would you please tell me your complaints?

P: I am having a very bad _____.

D: Oh. When did you experience the pain?

P: About six months ago but it was not so intense like what I felt last night. I felt pain at times and sometime it went off. But last night it got worse and even vomited blood.

D: OK. Can you show me where exactly the pain is?

P: It's here.

Patient is pointing to his upper abdomen – the epigastric region.

D: Can you tell me what the pain is like, is it dull pain or sharp pain? pricking or _____? Or hunger pain?

P: It's more like hunger pain, doctor.

D: Do you experience the pain continuously or it is intermittent?

P: Intermittent.

D: When do you feel the pain, before or after food?

P: It usually begins about 3 hours after meals then goes away after eating, but starts again 3 hours later.

D: Does this pain wake you up in the middle of your _____?

P: Yes. Early morning like 1:00 a.m. or 2:00 a.m. I have a pain and it goes away after eating some biscuit.

D: Is this first time you have vomited blood?

P: Yes. It is.

D: Do you remember the color of blood? Red or brown?

P: Yes, I do. It looked similar to grounded coffee.

D: Did you notice any _____ in the feces? Did the color change like brown or black?

P: No, Doctor. Nothing like that.

D: Did you experience fainting or chillness recently?

P: No. I felt little weak and tired.

D: OK, Mr. Wang, would you please take off your shirt and expose the abdomen so I can do some physical examination.

P: OK.

D: Now I am going to carry out the examination.

Doctor is palpating the epigastric region.

D: Do you feel the pain now? Is it radiating somewhere? Or do you feel pain anywhere else?

P: Yes, Doctor. It hurts and it is fixed here.

D: OK. Let me know if you have any pain.

Doctor withdraws his hand.

D: OK. Need to do some vital sign assessments. May I?

P: No Problem.

Doctor performs vital examination.

D: Mr. Wang, here is your vitals. Temp-36.8 ℃ , _____ 106/76 and Pulse-82. After careful considerations of your complaints and the examinations, you are suspected to have duodenal ulcer with complications of bleeding.

P：I got it. Doctor......

New Words & Expressions

throw up 呕吐   withdraw 收回，取回

bowel movement 大便   duodenal ulcer 十二指肠溃疡

emesis 呕吐

Passage

Answer the questions after listening to the passage.

1. Which one of the following organisms can cause ulcers?
A. Virus.   B. Bacteria.
C. Fungi.   D. Parasite.
2. What is the name of the drug that reduces acid production in the stomach?
A. Non-steroidal anti-inflammatory drugs.
B. Antibiotics.
C. Antacids.
D. Proton pump inhibitors.
3. What is the term peptic ulcer refers to?
A. Ulcer in the mouth.   B. Ulcer in the stomach.
C. Ulcer in the duodenum.   D. Both A and C.
4. All of the following can cause Peptic Ulcer EXCEPT
A. High dose of NSAIDs.   B. Long term use of NSAIDs.
C. Stress.   D. Bacterial infection.
5. Which one of the following is NOT the symptom of Gastric Ulcers?
A. Burning pain in the abdomen.   B. Indigestion.
C. Fever.   D. Heart burn.

Section B   Reading Comprehension

Text

A 34-year-old woman presents with painful, red "knots" on her right leg that appear to trace along her veins, which started 3-4 days ago. She denies any trauma, including venipuncture to this area. She also expresses concern about the general appearance of the skin on her arms, legs and trunk, which she states has looked "redder" for the last few years.

She has a complicated obstetric history, including one late-term miscarriage at 14 weeks' gestation, treated with dilation and curettage, and a subsequent pregnancy complicated by eclampsia, with the delivery of a healthy baby. She has not been started on any new medications. Her medical history is otherwise notable for a prior diagnosis of syphilis status post-antimicrobial therapy after a positive rapid plasma reagin (RPR) test.

A review of systems is notable for occasional subjective fevers and intermittent abdominal pain without any temporal relation to her meals, in addition to occasional pain and swelling of her knees and wrists. She denies any diarrhea or tarry or bloody stools.

Physical Examination and Workup

The patient is afebrile, with a temperature of 99.68°F (37.6°C). Her heart rate is 84 beats/min. Her respiratory rate is 12 breaths/min. Her blood pressure is 106/74mmHg. Her oxygen saturation is 97% on room air via pulse oximetry.

A physical examination is performed and is notable for several findings. Relating to her chief complaint, two red-to-purple, tender, indurated cords are observed on her right calf.

Also apparent on examination is a generalized, mottled, finely reticulated, violaceous discolouration of the skin on her arms, legs, and trunk. Punctuate to flame-shaped, subungual red markings can be appreciated on some of the nails of her hands and feet.

Inspection of the oral mucosa is revealing for an incidental finding of two, non-tender, punched-out ulcerations on the hard palate and left buccal mucosa. She has no appreciable cervical, axillary, or inguinal lymphadenopathy.

No obvious abnormalities are appreciated on cardiovascular examination. Her respirations are not labored, and lung fields are clear to auscultation. Her abdomen is soft, non-tender, and non-distended, with normal, active bowel sounds and no organomegaly.

Musculoskeletal examination is performed as well. Her right knee is mildly swollen and red, with range of motion only minimally limited due to pain. No other joint abnormalities are observed, despite her complaints. She has normal muscle bulk, tone, and strength.

Neurologic examination is largely unremarkable, with the exception of a mild, barely perceptible, facial asymmetry, which she reports having noticed suddenly a few months ago.

Venous duplex ultrasonography is performed and reveals the presence of a thrombus in the right leg, confirming the diagnosis of superficial thrombophlebitis. Radiography of the right knee shows no evidence of fracture, narrowing of the joint space, or articular degeneration.

Initial laboratory workup is performed. Complete blood count is significant for thrombocytopenia, elevated red cell distribution width, and a hypochromic, microcytic anemia with accompanying reticulocytosis and elevated serum lactate dehydrogenase. A comprehensive metabolic panel reveals no evidence of liver dysfunction but is revealing for an elevated serum creatinine level of 1.3 mg/dL. Coagulation studies demonstrate an abnormally prolonged activated partial thromboplastin time (APTT). Blood cultures and a herpes viral culture of her oral lesions have been ordered and are pending. Antinuclear antibody (ANA) titers are abnormally elevated, with follow-up serologic studies pending.

New Words & Expressions

venipuncture [ˌvenəˈpʌŋktʃə] *n.* the puncturing of a vein, esp to take a sample of venous blood or inject a drug 静脉穿刺

obstetric [əbˈstetrɪk] *a.* of or relating to childbirth 产科的；生产的；分娩的

miscarriage [mɪsˈkerɪdʒ] *n.* a natural loss of the products of conception 流产

dilation [daɪˈleɪʃ(ə)n] *n.* the act of expanding an aperture 扩张；扩大

eclampsia [ɪˈklæmpsiə] *n.* a toxic condition characterized by convulsions and possibly coma during or immediately after pregnancy 子痫；惊厥

syphilis [ˈsifəlis] *n.* a very serious disease that is passed from one person to another during sexual activity 梅毒

antimicrobial [ˌæntɪmaɪˈkrəʊbɪəl] *adj.* able to destroy harmful microbes [药] 抗菌的；杀菌的

tarry [ˈtæri] *a.* 柏油样的

oximetry [ɔkˈsimitri] *n.* a method to measure the oxygenated hemoglobin in the blood [临床] 血氧定量法

indurate [ˈɪndjʊəreɪt] *v.* make hard or harder 使硬化；使坚固

reticulate [rɪˈtɪkjəlɪt] *v.* form a net or a network 使……成网状的

violaceous [ˌvaɪəˈleɪʃəs] *a.* of, relating to, or belonging to the violaceae 紫罗兰色的

subungual [sjuːˈbʌŋjuːəl] *a.* 指甲下的

ulceration [ˌʌlsəˈreɪʃn] *n.* the development or formation of an ulcer 溃疡；[病理] 溃疡形成

axillary [æksɪləri] *a.* of, relating to, or near the armpit 腋窝的；靠近腋窝的

lymphadenopathy [lɪmˌfædəˈnɒpəθɪ] *n.* a swelling of the lymph nodes, usually caused by inflammation associated with a viral infection such as rubella 淋巴结病，肿大

asymmetry [ˌeɪˈsɪmətrɪ] *n.* the appearance that something has when its two sides or halves are different in shape, size, or style 不对称

thrombophlebitis [ˌθrɒmbəʊflɪˈbaɪtɪs] *n.* inflammation of a vein associated with the formation of a thrombus 血栓性静脉炎

thrombocytopenia [ˌθrɒmbəʊsaɪtəʊˈpiːnɪə] *n.* an abnormal decrease in the number of platelets in the blood 血小板减少

hypochromic [haɪpəʊˈkrəʊmɪk] *a.* 血红蛋白过少的

microcytic [ˌmaikrəʊˈsitik] *a.* 小红细胞性的；小红细胞的

reticulocytosis [rɪtɪkjʊləʊsaɪˈtəʊsɪs] *n.* 网状细胞过多症

dehydrogenase [ˌdiːˈhaɪdrədʒəneɪs] *n.* an enzyme, such as any of the respiratory enzymes, that activates oxidation-reduction reactions by transferring hydrogen from substrate to acceptor 脱氢酶

Exercise

Decide whether the following statements are true (T) or false (F) according to the passage.

_____1. The patient also expresses concern about the general appearance of the skin on her arms, legs, and trunk, which she states has looked "redder" for the last year.

_____2. A review of systems is notable for occasional subjective fevers and intermittent abdominal pain which is not temporally related the patient's meals.

_____3. There are some flame-shaped, subungual red markings on her nails of the patient's hands and feet.

_____4. The patient's abdomen is soft, non-tender, and swollen, with normal, active bowel sounds and no organomegaly.

_____5. Blood cultures and a herpes viral culture of the patient's oral lesions have been ordered but are not pending.

Answer the following questions according to the passage.

1. What obstetric history does the patient have?

_____

2. What is the most likely diagnosis that is causing this patient's superficial thrombophlebitis?

_____

3. What does a comprehensive metabolic panel reveal?

_____

Use the appropriate form of the words or phrases in the box to complete the following sentences.

asymmetry	plasma	miscarriage	trauma	ulceration
subungual	axillary	violaceous	syphilis	obstetric
venipuncture	non-tender	thrombophlebitis		

1. With no _____ risk, more women might be willing to take it, and so more women would find out they have a Down syndrome pregnancy.

2. Phlebitis can last for years, in such cases, irritation of the vein's inner lining leads to Blood-clot formation, a condition known as _____.

3. Diabetic foot problems are caused by changes in blood vessels and nerves that can lead to _____ and subsequent limb amputation.

4. Several, in particular HIV and _____, can also be transmitted from mother to child during pregnancy and childbirth, and through blood products and tissue transfer.

5. In order to give you intravenous infusion during your operation, now I'm giving you a _____ and a trocar in your vein.

6. It is noted that the information _____ between buyers and sellers caused insurance markets to malfunction.

7. As a result, more trained staffs have been recruited in district health centers in recent years and more pregnant women have gained access to essential _____ care.

8. _____ hematoma is a common injury after a blow or crush injury to the nail, which causes severe excruciating pain.

9. During this time, he fought in the Battle of Trenton, during which he was wounded by a bullet hitting his left shoulder and injuring the _____ artery, the major artery to his arm.

10. Our surgical tools allow us to operate on all parts of the body with a minimum of _____ and blood loss.

Translation

A. Translate the following expressions into English.

1. 血栓性浅静脉炎   2. 口腔病学
3. 腹股沟淋巴结病   4. 代谢功能检查
5. 柏油状或血便   6. 偶尔的发烧
7. 膝盖和手腕肿胀   8. 抗核抗体滴度

B. Translate the following sentences or expressions into Chinese.

1. A 34-year-old woman presents with painful, red "knots" on her right leg that appear to trace along her veins, which started 3-4 days ago.

2. Her medical history is otherwise notable for a prior diagnosis of syphilis status post-antimicrobial therapy after a positive rapid plasma reagin (RPR) test.

3. Also apparent on examination is a generalized, mottled, finely reticulated, violaceous discolouration of the skin on her arms, legs, and trunk.

4. Neurologic examination is largely unremarkable, with the exception of a mild, barely perceptible, facial asymmetry, which she reports having noticed suddenly a few months ago.

5. Complete blood count is significant for thrombocytopenia, elevated red cell distribution width, and a hypochromic, microcytic anemia with accompanying reticulocytosis and elevated serum lactate dehydrogenase.

Section C　Vocabulary (Terminology)

1. 消化 digestion

Combining form	Meaning	Terminology	Terminology meaning
-pepsia	digestion	dyspepsia	indigestion

2. 咽 throat

Combining form	Meaning	Terminology	Terminology meaning
pharyngo-	throat	pharyngeal	relating to or located or produced in the region of the pharynx 咽的

3. 食管 esophagus

Combining form	Meaning	Terminology	Terminology meaning
esophago-	esophagus	esophagitis	inflammation of the esophagus 食管炎

4. 胃 stomach

Combining form	Meaning	Terminology	Terminology meaning
gastro-	stomach	gastrectomy	surgical removal of all or part of the stomach 胃切除术

5. 肠 intestine, bowel, gut

Combining form	Meaning	Terminology	Terminology meaning
entero-	Intestine, usually small intestine	enterocolitis	enteritis affecting both the large and small intestine 大小肠炎

6. 十二指肠 duodenum

Combining form	Meaning	Terminology	Terminology meaning
duodeno-	duodenum	duodenoscopy	十二指肠镜检查

7. 空肠 jejunum

Combining form	Meaning	Terminology	Terminology meaning
jejuno-	jejunum	gastrojejunostomy	胃空肠吻合术

8. 回肠 ileum

Combining form	Meaning	Terminology	Terminology meaning
ileo-	ileum	ileitis	inflammation of the ileum 回肠炎

9. 结肠 colon

Combining form	Meaning	Terminology	Terminology meaning
colo-	colon,	colitis	inflammation of the colon 结肠炎
colono-	colon	colonoscopy	endoscopic examination of the colon 结肠镜检查

10. 盲肠 cecum

Combining form	Meaning	Terminology	Terminology meaning
ceco-	cecum	cecal	of or relating cecum 盲肠的

11. 阑尾 appendix

Combining form	Meaning	Terminology	Terminology meaning
appendo-	appendix	appendectomy	surgical removal of the vermiform appendix 阑尾切除手术
appendico-	appendix	appendicitis	inflammation of the vermiform appendix 阑尾炎

12. 乙状结肠 sigmoid

Combining form	Meaning	Terminology	Terminology meaning
sigmoido-	sigmoid	sigmoidoscopy	an endoscope designed to be passed through the anus for visual examination especially of the sigmoid colon 乙状结肠镜检查

13. 直肠 rectum

Combining form	Meaning	Terminology	Terminology meaning
recto-	rectum	rectocele	直肠突出
procto-	anus and rectum	proctoscopy	直肠镜检查

14. 肛门 aus

Combining form	Meaning	Terminology	Terminology meaning
ano-	anus	anorectitis	肛门直肠炎

15. 肝 liver

Combining form	Meaning	Terminology	Terminology meaning
hepato-	liver	hepatomegaly	enlargement of the liver 肝肿大

16. 胆囊 gallbladder

Combining form	Meaning	Terminology	Terminology meaning
cholecysto-	gallbladder	cholecystitis	inflammation of the gallbladder 胆囊炎

17. 胆总管 common bile duct

Combining form	Meaning	Terminology	Terminology meaning
choledocho-	common bile duct	choledocholith	胆总管结石

18. 胆管 bile duct

Combining form	Meaning	Terminology	Terminology meaning
cholangio-	bile duct	cholangiography	radiographic visualization of the bile ducts after injection of a radiopaque substance 胆管造影术

19. 胰腺 pancreas

Combining form	Meaning	Terminology	Terminology meaning
pancreato-	pancreas	pancreatitis	inflammation of the pancreas 胰腺炎

20. 脸 face

Combining form	Meaning	Terminology	Terminology meaning
facio-	face	facial	of or relating to face 脸的

21. 颊 cheek

Combining form	Meaning	Terminology	Terminology meaning
bucco-	cheek	buccal mucosa	a mucosa is composed of epithelial cells 颊的

22. 下颌骨 lower jaw, mandible

Combining form	Meaning	Terminology	Terminology meaning
mandibulo-	lower jaw, mandible	submandibular	of, relating to, situated in, or performed in the region below the lower jaw 下颌下的

23. 唇 lip

Combining form	Meaning	Terminology	Terminology meaning
cheilo-	lip	cheilosis	唇干裂
labio	lip	labial	of or relating to lips 唇的

24. 口 mouth

Combining form	Meaning	Terminology	Terminology meaning
or/o	mouth	oral	of, given through, or involving the mouth 口的
stomat/o	mouth	stomatitis	any of numerous inflammatory diseases of the mouth 口炎

25. 牙齿 tooth

Combining form	Meaning	Terminology	Terminology meaning
denti-	tooth	dentin	a calcareous material similar to but harder and denser than bone that composes the principal mass of a tooth 牙质
odonto-	tooth	endodontist	a branch of dentistry concerned with diseases of the pulp 牙髓病学家

26. 牙龈 gum

Combining form	Meaning	Terminology	Terminology meaning
gingivo-	gum	gingivitis	inflammation of the gums 牙龈炎

27. 舌 tongue

Combining form	Meaning	Terminology	Terminology meaning
glosso	tongue	hypoglossal	situated or administered under the tongue 舌下的
linguo	tongue	sublingual	situated or administered under the tongue 舌下的

28. 腭 palate

Combining form	Meaning	Terminology	Terminology meaning
palato-	palate	palatoplasty	the procedure corrects cleft (split) palate, a congenital anomaly 腭成形术

29. 腹 belly, abdomen

Combining form	Meaning	Terminology	Terminology meaning
celio-	belly,abdomen	celiac	of or relating to the abdominal cavity 腹腔的
abdomino-	belly,abdomen	abdominocentesis	a tube is placed through an incision of the abdomen and fluid is removed from peritoneal cavity 腹腔穿刺
laparo-	belly,abdomen	laparoscopy	visual examination of the abdomen by means of a laparoscope 腹腔镜检查

30. 腹膜 peritoneum

Combining form	Meaning	Terminology	Terminology meaning
periton(eo)	peritoneum	peritonitis	inflammation of the peritoneum 腹膜炎

31. 淀粉 starch

Combining form	Meaning	Terminology	Terminology meaning
amyl/o	starch	amylase	any of a group of enzymes (as amylopsin) that catalyze the hydrolysis of starch and glycogen or their intermediate hydrolysis products 淀粉酶

32. 胆汁 bile, gall

Combining form	Meaning	Terminology	Terminology meaning
bil/i	gall, bile	biliary	of, relating to, or conveying bile 胆汁的，胆的
chol/e	gall, bile	cholelithiasis	production of gallstones 胆石症

33. 胆红素 bilirubin

Combining form	Meaning	Terminology	Terminology meaning
bilirubin/o	bilirubin bile pigment	hyperbilirubinemia	high level of bilirubin in the blood 高胆红素血症

34. 盐酸 hydrochloric acid

Combining form	Meaning	Terminology	Terminology meaning
chlorhydr/o	hydrochloric acid	achlorhydria	absence of hydrochloric acid from the gastric juice 胃酸缺乏症

35. 糖 sugar

Combining form	Meaning	Terminology	Terminology meaning
gluc/o	sugar	gluconeogensis	liver cells make new sugar from fats and proteins 动物淀粉新生
glyc/o	sugar	hyperglycemia	hyperglycemia 血糖过高症

36. 糖原 glycogen

Combining form	Meaning	Terminology	Terminology meaning
glycogen/o	glycogen, animal starch	glycogenolysis	the breakdown of glycogen especially to glucose in the animal body 糖原分解

37. 脂肪（类）fat, lipid

Combining form	Meaning	Terminology	Terminology meaning
lip/o	fat, lipid	lipoma	a tumor of fatty tissue 脂肪瘤
steato	fat	steatorrhea	an excess of fat in the stools 脂肪痢

38. 结石 calculus, stone

Combining form	Meaning	Terminology	Terminology meaning
lith/o	stone	cholelithiasis	production of gallstones 胆石症

39. 酶 enzyme

Combining form	Meaning	Terminology	Terminology meaning
-ase	enzyme	lipase	an enzyme that hydrolyzes glycerides 脂酶

40. 大便 defecation

Combining form	Meaning	Terminology	Terminology meaning
-chezia	defecation, elimination of wastes	hematochezia	bright red blood is found in the feces.

41. 异常 abnormal condition

Combining form	Meaning	Terminology	Terminology meaning
-iasis	abnormal condition	cholelithiasis	production of gallstones 胆石症

Exercise for vocabulary

Write down the meaning of the given combining forms in English.

1. lith/o means _____
2. -chezia means _____
3. -iasis means _____
4. lapar/o means _____
5. hepat/o means _____
6. gastr/o means _____
7. choledoch/o means _____
8. appendic/o means _____
9. enter/o means _____
10. col/o means _____
11. esophag/o means _____
12. ile/o means _____
13. pancreat/o means _____
14. peritone/o means _____
15. amyl/o means _____
16. gluc/o means _____
17. lip/o means _____
18. bilirubin/o means _____
19. bil/I means _____
20. cholecyst/o means _____

Match the following terms with their meaning below.

hyperglycemia	hyperbilirubinemia	cholangiography	dysphagia
laparoscopy	cholecystitis	amylase	appendicitis
glycogenolysis	hepatomegaly		

_____1. High level of blood sugar

_____2. Any of a group of enzymes (as amylopsin) that catalyze the hydrolysis of starch and glycogen or their intermediate hydrolysis products

_____3. Enlargement of the liver

_____4. Visual examination of the abdomen by means of a laparoscope

_____5. Inflammation of the gallbladder

_____6. Inflammation of the vermiform appendix

_____7. Radiographic visualization of the bile ducts after injection of a radiopaque substance

_____8. High level of bilirubin in the blood

_____9. Difficulty in swallowing

_____10. The breakdown of glycogen especially to glucose in the animal body

Fill in the blank with the words given below.

gastroenterologist	disease	inflammatory	bowel	odynophagia
gingivitis	pancratitis	gastroesophageal	reflux	dysmenorrhea
cirrhosis	hepatitis	platoplasty		

1. When Mrs. Smith developed diarrhea and cramp abdominal pain, she consulted a _____ and worried that she might have _____.

2. After taking a careful history and physical, Dr. Blakemore diagnosed Mr. Bean, a long-time drinker, with _____. Mr. Bean had complained of sharp midepigastric pain and a change in bowel habits.

3. Many pregnant women cannot lie flat after eating because of a burning sensation in their chest and throat. Doctors call this condition _____.

4. Pediatric surgeon must be wary of _____ in young infants who display projectile vomiting.

5. Boris had terrible problems with his teeth. He needed not only a periodontitis for his _____ but also an orthodontist to straight his teeth.

6. After six weeks of radiation therapy to her throat, Betty experienced severe esophageal irritation and inflammation. She complained to her doctor about her.

7. Barbara had cramping and bloating before otherwise normal menstrual periods. Her physician prescribed pain medication to alleviate her.

8. Chris had been a heavy alcohol drinker all of his adult life. His wife gradually noticed yellow discolouration of the whites of his eyes and skin. After a physical examination and blood tests, his family physician told him his liver was diseased. The yellow discolouration was jaundice and his condition was _____.

9. When Carol had been a phlebotomist, she accidentally cut her finger while drawing a patient's blood. Unfortunately, the patient had _____ and HBV was transmitted to Carol. Blood test and liver biopsy confirmed Carol's unfortunate diagnosis. The doctor told her that her condition was chronic and that she might be a candidate for a liver transplant in the future.

10. Operation Smile is a rescue project that performs _____ on children with a congenital cleft in the roof of their mouth.

Section D   Writing

Chief Complaints

我们在上一章介绍了一般项目的英文写法，我们现在来讲述一下主诉的写作。在我国，主诉的写法要求简明精练，一般为 1 ～ 2 句，20 字左右，其内容包括症状、体征及持续时间。主诉多于一项则按时间的先后次序列出，并记录每个症状的持续时间。而英文的主诉通常包括以下内容：患者的年龄，简要的相关既往病史，寥寥数语阐述患者来院诊治的原因（最好引用患者的原话，并用引号表示），最后陈述目前症状持续的时间。全部这些内容必须控制在 2 行之内。

Example 1: A 57-year-old woman presents to the ED with a 3-day history of colicky lower abdominal pain and diarrhea.

例 1：某某，女，57 岁，因下腹绞痛并腹泻 3 天入急诊科就诊。

Example 2: A 61-year-old woman with HIV infection and a CD4+ T-lymphocyte count of 280 cells per cubic millimeter presents with a fever, pharyngitis, and dysphagia that have lasted 3 days.

例 2：某某，女，61 岁，感染艾滋病，其 CD4+T 淋巴细胞计数 280 个 /mm³，主诉发热，咽炎，吞咽困难 3 天。

Example 3: 56-year-old male with a history of ulcerative colitis complaining of 3 months of worsening back stiffness, 2 weeks of "a sore on my leg", and 3 days of fevers and bloody, painless diarrhea.

例 3：某某，男，56 岁，曾患溃疡性结肠炎，主诉背部僵直逐渐加重 3 月，"肢体疼痛" 2 周，发热、无痛性血便 3 天。

从上例我们可以看出 chief complaints 一般由症状和持续时间两部分构成，主要有以下几种写法：

1. 症状 + for + 时间（这种用得最多）

Example 4: A 22-year-old previously healthy woman presents to the emergency department with acute shortness of breath for 2 days.

例 4：某某，女，22 岁，既往健康，因急性气短 32 天而入急诊科就诊。

2. 症状 + of + 时间 + duration

Example 5: A 23-year-old woman presented to the emergency department with diffuse, colicky abdominal pain of 1 hour's duration.

例 5：某某，女，23 岁，因弥漫性腹部绞痛 1 小时而入急诊科就诊。

3. 症状 + 时间 + for + 时间 + duration

Example 6: A 38-year-old male patient was admitted on August, 11, 2018 complaining of right upper abdominal pain for 17 hours' duration.

例 6：某某，男，38 岁因右上腹疼痛 17 小时于 2018 年 8 月 11 日入院。

4. 时间 + of + 症状

Example 7: 27-year-old man came to the emergency department because of a 2-day history of fever, headache, and general malaise.

例 7：某某，男，27 岁因发热、头痛、全身不适 2 天来急诊科就诊。

5. 症状 + 时间 + in duration

Example 8: A 42-year-old male was admitted on July, 1st, 2017, complaining of vomiting 3 days in duration.

例 8：某某，男，42 岁因呕吐 3 天于 2017 年 7 月 1 日入院。

6. 症状 + since + 症状开始的时间点

Example 9: A 28-year-old married female was admitted to hospital on August, 5th, 2018 for because of vaginal bleeding since yesterday.

例 9：某某，女，28 岁，已婚，于 2018 年 8 月 5 日因自昨天阴道出血入院。

7. 时间段（合成词）+ history of + 症状

Example 10: A 60-year-old man presents to the ED with a 1-day history of left-sided abdominal pain.

例 10：某某，男，60 岁，因左腹疼痛 1 天于急诊科就诊。

常见句式：

主诉部分，在住院病历或门诊病历中，常用省略句。然而，在首次病程记录（住院记录）中，主诉要用完整句来描述。常用的有下面几种。

1. was admitted to hospital on month/date/year complaining of

Example 11: A 21-year-old woman was admitted on July, 17th, 2018 complaining of a 1-month history of fever, general malaise, and mild diffuse and cramping abdominal pain.

例 11：某某，女，21 岁因发热，全身不适及轻度弥漫性痉挛性腹痛 1 月于 2018 年 7 月 17 日入院。

2. present to ED/your office with …

Example 12: A 57-year-old woman presents to the ED with a 3-day history of colicky lower abdominal pain and diarrhea.

例 12：某某，女，57 岁，因下腹部绞痛及泄泻 3 天于急诊科就诊。

3. complain of …

Example 13: the patient, an unmarried adult female, complained of a 6-year intermittent abdominalgia which has been worsening in the last 3 days.

例 13：某某，未婚成年女性，主诉间歇性腹痛 6 年加重 3 天。

4. was admitted … because of

Example 14: A 28-year-old married female was admitted to the hospital on May, 3rd, 2018 because of a 6-day fever and cough.

例 14：某某，28 岁，女性，已婚，因发热咳嗽 6 天，于 2018 年 5 月 3 日入院。

5. was referred to … because of

Example 15: The 32-year-old married female with history of nephrotic syndrome was referred to the digestive department because of ascites.

例 15：某某，女，32 岁，因肾病综合征腹水转诊于消化科。

实例：

例 16：

主诉：突起畏寒、高热伴咳嗽、胸痛 2 天

Example 16:

CC (chief complaint): sudden onset of cold intolerance and high fever with 2-day history of cough and chest pain.

例 17：

主诉：反复咳嗽咳痰 10 余年，气促 5 年加重 1 天。

Example 17:

CC (chief complaint): recurrent productive cough over 10 years and tachypnea 5 year which have been worsening 1 day.

例 18：

主诉：某某，男，50 岁，因慢性咳嗽、咳痰 10 余年，加重伴发热 1 周于 2017 年 12 月 26 日入院。

Example 18:

A 50-year-old male was admitted to hospital on Dec, 26th, 2017 because of chronic productive cough more than 10 years which has been worsening with fever for 1 week.

Exercise

Directions: translate the following chief complaints into English.

1. 某某，女，60 岁，慢性肺心病患者，因上腹胀、尿少、全身浮肿 1 天于 2007 年 1 月 16 日入院。

2. 主诉：心悸气促 10 年，加重 3 天。

3. 主诉：突起心悸气促，咳粉红色泡沫痰。

4. 主诉：胸骨后疼痛伴反胃 2 年。

5. 主诉：上腹部不适 5 年，早饱、嗳气 1 月。

6. 某某，女，28 岁，腹胀、腹痛 6 月，加重伴发热 2 周于 2018 年 4 月 2 日入院。

7. 感冒 5 天后出现面部及双下肢浮肿、尿少。

8. 某某，女，24 岁，因突发寒战、高热、腰痛、尿急、尿频、尿痛于 2008 年 3 月 22 日入院。

Section E   Spoken English

Role play

Directions: 3 students are selected to demonstrate the conversation, one plays the role of Attending Dr. Zeng, another plays the role of Resident Dr. Liu, the last one plays the role of Resident Dr. Zhang, they are discussing about a case of portal cirrhosis with ascites ......

Discussion

Directions: Work in groups and discuss with your partners, then answer the following questions with detailed analysis.

Mr. Donaldson, 47-year-old, was presented to the emergency department with a 12-hour history of vomiting bright red blood. He has had 4 episodes of emesis during this time span. He also complained of nausea, fatigue, and lightheadedness. He had 1 episode of melena shortly before arrival. He denied abdominal pain, diarrhea, or fever. He has a history of hypertension and chronic back pain from a car accident. His medications include hydrochlorothiazide, amlodipine, and ibuprofen. He smokes 1 pack per day. He also drinks 6 to 8 cans of beer per day, with more on the weekends and holidays. He has drunk this amount of alcohol for 22 years. On examination, he appears drowsy, with a blood pressure of 94/46 mm Hg, heart rate of 122 bpm, respiratory rate of 24 breaths/min, and oxygen saturation of 96% on room air. He is afebrile. His eyes are slightly icteric. His oral mucosa is slightly dry. Chest auscultation reveals clear lungs and a regular heart rhythm. Abdominal examination reveals mild distention and evidence of hepatomegaly. His rectal examination reveals heme-positive stool.

Laboratory data show hemoglobin 9.8, hematocrit 29, and platelets 98,000. BUN is 28 and creatinine is 1.2. INR is 1.6. AST is 102 and ALT is 68.

1. What is the most likely diagnosis?

2. What is the initial goal of evaluation and patient care?

3. What else is on the differential diagnosis?

Terminology related to gastrointestinal department

gastritis 胃炎

acute gastritis 急性胃炎

chronic gastritis 慢性胃炎

acute diarrhea 急性腹泻

acute liver failure 急性肝衰竭

acute pancreatitis 急性胰腺炎

acute viral hepatitis 急性肝炎

appendicitis 阑尾炎

ascites 腹水

Barrett's esophagus Barrett 食管

bile acid 胆汁酸

carcinoma of the esophagus 食管癌

carcinoma of the colon 结肠癌

carcinoma of the rectum 直肠癌

carcinoma of the pancreas 胰腺癌

cholangitis 胆管炎

cholecystitis 胆囊炎

cholelithiasis 胆石症

chronic diarrhea 慢性腹泻

cirrhosis of liver 肝硬化

colitis 结肠炎

intestinal obstruction 肠梗阻

ileus 肠梗阻

colon ischemia 结肠缺血

colonoscopy 肠镜检查术

constipation 便秘

colon cancer 结肠癌

complication 并发症

Crohn's disease 克罗恩病

diarrhea 腹泻

diverticulitis 憩室炎

duodenal ulcer 十二指肠溃疡

dyspepsia 消化不良

dyschezia 大便困难

dysphagia 吞咽困难

endoscopy 内视镜检查法

esophagitis 食管炎

enteritis 肠炎

flapping tremor 扑翼性震颤

functional dyspepsia 功能性消化不良

fulminant hepatitis 暴发性肝炎

gallstone 胆结石

gastric cancer 胃癌

gastric ulcer 胃溃疡

gastric polyps 胃息肉

gastric perforation 胃穿孔

gastroenteritis 肠胃炎

gastroesophageal reflux disease 反流性胃食管疾病

gastrointestinal bleeding 胃肠出血

gastroesophageal varices 胃食管曲张

Gilbert syndrome 吉伯特综合征

H2-receptor blocking agents H2 受体阻滞剂

hemorrhoid 痔疮

hepatic encephalopathy 肝性脑病

hepatic jaundice 肝性黄疸

hepatic coma 肝性昏迷

hepatitis 肝炎

Hepatitis B 乙型肝炎

hepatocellular carcinomas 肝细胞癌

hyperbilirirubinemia 高胆红素血症

hepatorenal syndrome 肝肾综合征

hepatojugular reflux 肝颈静脉回流征

hepatosplenomegaly 肝脾肿大

hypertriblyceridemia 高甘油三酯血症

ileus 肠梗阻

incontinence 二便失禁

intestinal tuberculosis 肠结核

intrahepatic cholestatic jaundice 肝内胆汁淤积性黄疸

irritable bowel syndrome 肠易激综合征

liver abscess 肝脓肿

liver failure 肝功能衰竭

liver palm 肝掌

liver transplantation 肝移植

malaria 疟疾

malignant ascite 恶性腹腔积液

melena 黑粪症

peptic ulcer 消化性溃疡

percussion tenderness over hepatic region 肝区叩击痛

primary carcinoma of the liver 原发性肝癌

regurgitation 反酸

rebound tenderness 反跳痛

serum total protein 血清总蛋白

albumin 白蛋白

globulin 球蛋白

serum total bilirubin 血清总胆红素

alanine aminotransferase (ALT) 丙氨酸基转移酶

aspartate aminotransferase (AST) 天门冬氨基转移酶

Hepatitis B virus surface antigen 乙肝表面抗原

Hepatitis B virus surface antibody 乙肝表面抗体

Hepatitis B virus e antigen 乙肝 e 抗原

Hepatitis B virus e antibody 乙肝 e 抗体

Hepatitis B virus core antigen 乙肝核心抗原

Hepatitis B virus core antibody 乙肝核心抗体

urea nitrogen 尿素氮

alkaline phosphatase 碱性磷酸酶

direct bilirubin 直接胆红素

indirect bilirubin 非直接胆红素

prothrombin time 凝血酶原时间

thrombin time 凝血酶时间

serum amino 血氨

cholesterol 胆固醇

free bilirubin 游离胆红素

conjugated bilirubin 结合胆红素

unconjugated bilirubin 非结合胆红素

spider angioma 蜘蛛痣

tuberculous peritonitis 结核性腹膜炎

upper gastrointestinal bleeding 上消化道出血

ulcerative colitis 溃疡性结肠炎

urobilinogen 尿胆原

peritoneal irritation sign 腹膜刺激征

tenderness 压痛

rebound tenderness 反跳痛

liver thrill 肝震颤

Murphy sign 墨菲征

fluid thrill 液波震颤

fluctuation　波动感

succession splash　振水音

shifting dullness　移动性浊音

gurgling sound　肠鸣音

Rovsing sign　罗夫辛氏征

abdominal retraction　腹部凹陷

abdominal bulge　腹部

proctopolypus　直肠息肉

proctoptosis　直肠脱垂

hedrocele　脱肛

archosyrinx　肛瘘

hemorrhoid　痔疮

internal hemorrhoid　内痔

external hemorrhoid　外痔

mixed hemorrhoid　混合痔

anal fissure　肛裂

Chapter 5

Kidney and Urinary System

Section A   Focus Listening

Listen to the dialogue and fill in the blanks with proper words.

D= doctor P=patient

D: Chief Dr. Xie, your friend from respiratory department, asked me to have a word with you. Except the _____ symptoms you're having, what other symptoms do you have?

P: Oh, Doctor, I have to run back and forth to the toilet to pass water all the time, and it burns and stings every time.

D: How often does this happen? All the time or just intermittently?

P: It worsens or eases. When I get a bout of _____, the symptoms are worsened, it can last for about one week. I can't stand it. You know how embarrassing it is to run back and forth to the toilet. When I don't get a bout of infection, the symptoms are alleviated, I can live with it.

D: Can you describe the water work?

P: Well, this bout began yesterday, I've been having trouble getting started, it's painful and urgent.

D: Have you noticed any blood or discoloration in your urine?

P: Yes, I found blood in the urine this morning.

D: Does anything special bring it on?

P: I found that it attacked me after I had intercourse with my husband.

D: Was it brown color at that time?

P: Yes, it was.

D: How is your health otherwise, apart from this? Do you have diabetes, heart disease or blood pressure?

P: No.

D: Are you on any other _____?

P: No, I don't take any medication currently, I think I'm healthy.

D: Now I'd like to examine your abdomen, then we will do some tests for you. Please get undressed so that I can see your abdomen. Would you please lie down on the bed and I'll come around and examine you?

P: I'm ready, Doctor.

D: Does it hurt when I press on the suprapubic region?

P: Ouch! Yeah, yeah, it hurts badly.

D: OK, you can get down now, here are some test sheets. Firstly, you need send some your urine _____ to the laboratory to check whether there's any infection present. Secondly, I strongly advise you in the meantime to drink plenty of water because I will organize an ultrasound scan to assess the renal tract further. At last, please come back here, I'll prescribe some medications.

P: OK, is it serious, do I need take admission for treatment?

D: Nope, it can be cured in 3-5 days with proper treatment.

About half an hour later, the patient came back with test results.

D: The ultrasound reveals that you have acute _____. The urinalysis shows: protein positive. I'll prescribe antibiotics for you.

New Words & Expressions

pass water 解小便   suprapubic 耻骨上弓的
sting 刺痛   antibiotic 抗生素
diabetes 糖尿病

Passage

Answer the questions after listening to the passage.

1. Which one of the following substances is NOT a renal stone?

A. Urea.   B. Uric Acid.

C. Calcium Oxalate.   D. Struvite.

2. What is the most common age group to develop renal stones?

A. Between 10 and 20 years.   B. Between 20 and 40 years.

C. Between 50 and 60 years.   D. Above 60 years.

3. Which one of the following substances forms Randall's Plaque?

A. Struvite.   B. Uric acid.

C. Calcium oxalate.   D. Cystine.

4. Which one of the following is classical symptom of Renal Colic?

A. Fever.

B. Vomiting

C. Headache.

D. Sudden severe pain.

5. Which one of the following is true regarding the size of the renal stones?

A. They usually vary in size.

B. They are usually smaller in size.

C. They are usually larger in size.

D. None of the above.

Section B　Reading Comprehension

Text

A 68-year-old woman was admitted to the hospital because of impaired renal function. One month earlier, she had difficulty in breathing and felt as though she had a fever, she went to a hospital, where nebulizers were prescribed, and her dyspnea was improved. Two weeks later, malaise and a sensation of chilliness developed, with diffuse pains in the arms and legs, which prompted her to take two or three tablets of ibuprofen every four to five hours for two weeks, although the medication was only minimally effective. Ten days before admission, pruritus developed. She consulted a physician, who found that her temperature was 37.8℃ and prescribed cetirizine.

Four days later, she consulted her customary physician. The urine was ++ for protein; the sediment contained 50 to 100 white cells and moderate numbers of tubular cells. The urea nitrogen level was 20 mg per deciliter (7.1 mmol per liter), and the creatinine level 1.5 mg per deciliter (132.6 μmol per liter), although previously, the creatinine level had been around 0.8 mg per deciliter (70.7 μmol per liter). She was advised to discontinue taking ibuprofen and to return for follow-up, but on the day of admission she vomited twice, felt extremely fatigued, continued to have malaise, and produced less urine than usual. She was admitted to the hospital.

The patient had a history of hypertension. Six years before admission, she had had an abdominal hysterectomy with incidental appendectomy because of endometrial carcinoma. She had smoked one pack of cigarettes daily for 20 years but had stopped smoking 30 years before admission. She consumed wine with dinner. She resided with her husband and had several children, one of whom had multiple sclerosis. Her medications were hydrochlorothiazide, conjugated equine estrogens, aspirin, and a multivitamin tablet, as well as ibuprofen. She had no recurrence of dyspnea or fever, and she reported not having had frank chills, chest pain, abdominal pain, diarrhea, dysuria, polyuria, arthralgia, or rash or having recently traveled.

The temperature was 37.3℃, the pulse 66 beats per minute, and the respiratory rate 20 breaths per minute. The blood pressure was 110/75 mmHg. The oxygen saturation was 99 percent while the patient breathed ambient air. On physical examination, there was no rash or lymphadenopathy, and no petechiae were found. The jugular venous pressure was 7 cm of blood. The lungs were clear, and the heart sounds were normal. The abdomen was unremarkable. There was trace peripheral edema, and the pulses at the hands and feet were intact.

The urine was +++ for protein, had a specific gravity above 1.030, and was trace positive for ketones; the sediment contained 0 to 2 red and white cells, moderate numbers of squamous and transitional cells, and a few bacteria per high-power field and contained 0 to 2 hyaline casts, 3 to 5 granular casts, and 0 to 2 waxy casts per low-power field. The results of hematologic and other laboratory tests performed on admission are reported in Table 1 and Table 2, respectively. An electrocardiogram showed a normal rhythm at a rate of 65 beats per minute, with a corrected QT interval of 487 milliseconds and minor ST-segment and T-wave abnormalities.

Table 1. Hematologic Laboratory Data on Admission

Variable	Value
Hematocrit (%)	37.2
White-cell count (Per mm^3)	14,700
Differential count (%)	
neutrophils	66
lymphocytes	11
Atypical lymphocytes	1
Bands	4
Monocytes	4
Eosinophils	14
platelets (Per mm^3)	208,000
Mean corpuscular volume (μm^3)	87
Prothrombin time	Normal
Partial-thromboplastin time	Normal

Table 2. Blood Chemical Values

Variable	On admission	2nd hospital day	3rd hospital day	4th hospital day	5th hospital day
Glucose	Normal				
bilirubin					
Conjugated	Normal				
Total	Normal				

续表

Variable	On admission	2nd hospital day	3rd hospital day	4th hospital day	5th hospital day
Phosphorus(mg/dl)	6.3				16.1
Protein(g/dl)	7.4				
Albumin	2.0				
Globulin	5.4				
Cholesterol(mg/dl)			181		
High-density lipoprotein			22		
Low-density lipoprotein			98		
triglyceride(mg/dl)			307		
Sodium(mmol/liter)	125		120	124	124
Potassium(mmol/liter)	3.0		3.3	3.6	4.3
Chloride(mmol/liter)	95		86	81	83
Carbon dioxide (mmol/liter)	24.5		20.8	14.9	17.6
Magnesium(mmol/liter)	Normal				1.0
Urea nitrogen(mg/dl)	40	43	63	80	98
Creatinine(mg/dl)	3.7	4.0	6.2	7.2	7.6
calcium(mg/dl)	7.1				5.6
Creatinine kinase	Normal				
Creatinine kinase isoenzymes	Normal				
Troponin T	Normal				
Alkaline phosphatase	Normal				
Aspartate aminotransferase (U/liter)	66				
Alanine aminotrasferase (U/liter)	51				
Amylase	Normal				
lipase	Normal				
IgG(mg/dl)		1980			
IgA(mg/dl)		506			
IgM(mg/dl)		Normal			
C4(mg/dl)		15			
Test for antinuclear antibodies		Positive (at 1:40 and 1:160), with a speckled pattern			
Serum protein electrophoresis		Abnormal 2 very low concentration bands in slow gamma region, identified as IgG kappa M components			

An abdominopelvic computed tomographic (CT) study revealed a small amount of pericardial thickening or fluid and minimal atelectasis at the base of the left lung; no hydronephrosis was observed. The right kidney was unremarkable, and the left contained a calcification, 2 mm in diameter, which was consistent with the presence of a calculus. The urine-collecting systems and bladder were normal. There were diverticula in the sigmoid colon, but they were not inflamed. A low-attenuation lesion within the dome of the liver and another in the right hepatic lobe were unchanged relative to a study performed 18 months earlier. Several sub-centimeter lymph nodes were seen in the paraaortic region, and one was seen in the right external iliac chain; several prominent inguinal nodes were noted bilaterally. The stomach, small bowel, and skeletal structures were normal. Chest radiographs showed stable thickening of the apical pleura bilaterally; the lungs, heart, mediastinum, and bony thorax were normal.

Ibuprofen and hydrochlorothiazide were discontinued, and intravenous administration of nonessential fluids was avoided. Morphine was provided for pain and lorazepam for sleeplessness, and the administration of low dosage of heparin was begun. The patient was afebrile at all times.

On the second hospital day, her pruritus and nausea resolved, and she felt much improved. The urinary volume was 80 to 90 ml during each eight-hour shift. The results of laboratory tests performed that day are shown in Table 2. No Bence Jones protein was detected; the urine contained a large amount of albumin, a small amount of α-globulin, a moderate amount of β-globulin, and a moderate amount of probably intact immunoglobulin. The total urinary protein excretion was 3.4 g per 24 hours.

On the third hospital day, the patient continued to feel well. Physical examination revealed no abnormalities except for trace peripheral edema. Intravenous administration of methylprednisolone (500 mg daily) was begun. During the next two days, the patient remained comfortable. The results of laboratory tests performed from the third day to the fifth day are shown in Table 2. The oliguria persisted. Culture specimens of blood and urine were sterile.

A diagnostic procedure was performed on the fifth hospital day.

New Words & Expressions

nebulizer ['nebjulaizə] *n.* a dispenser that turns a liquid (such as perfume)into a fine mist [分化] 喷雾器

dyspnea [dɪsp'niə] *n.* difficult or labored respiration [内科] 呼吸困难

malaise [mə'leɪz] *n.* physical discomfort (as mild sickness or depression) 不舒服；心神不安

ibuprofen [ˌaɪbjuː'prəʊfen] *n.* a medicine that reduces pain, inflammation, and fever

布洛芬

pruritus [prʊˈraɪtəs] *n*. [皮肤] 瘙痒，瘙痒症

hysterectomy [ˌhɪstəˈrektəmi] *n*. a medical operation to remove a woman's uterus 子宫切除（术）

endometrial [endʌˈmetrɪəl] *a*. of or relating to the endometrium [解剖] 子宫内膜的

hydrochlorothiazide [ˈhaɪdrəʊˌklɔːrəˈθaɪəzaɪd] *n*. 氢氯噻嗪；二氢氯噻

petechiae [pəˈtekɪeɪ] *n*. 瘀点，出血

peripheral [pəˈrɪfərəl] *a*. on or near an edge or constituting an outer boundary;the outer area 外围的；次要的；（神经）末梢区域的

hematologic [ˌheməˈtɒlədʒɪk] *a*. of or relating to or involved in hematology 血液学的

atelectasis [ˌætəˈlektəsɪs] *n*. 肺不张；（出生时肺的）膨胀不全

hydronephrosis [ˌhaɪdrənɪˈfrəʊsɪs] *n*. accumulation of urine in the kidney because of an obstruction in the ureter [病理学] 肾盂积水

diverticula [daɪvəˈtikjulə] *n*. 憩室（ diverticulum 的复数 ）

inguinal [ˈɪŋgwɪnəl] *a*. of or relating to the groin [解剖][动] 腹股沟的；鼠蹊部的

afebrile [eɪˈfiːbraɪl] *a*. having no fever 无热的

immunoglobulin [ɪˈmjuːnəʊˈglɒbjʊlɪn] *n*. 免疫球蛋白；免疫血球素

oliguria [ɒlɪˈgjʊərɪə] *n*. abnormally small production of urine 少尿，尿过少

Exercise

Decide whether the following statements are true (T) or false (F) according to the passage.

_____1. The patient had difficulty breathing and a fever one month ago, then she went to one hospital, where nebulizers were prescribed, but her dyspnea wasn't improved.

_____2. When the patient consulted her customary physician, her urine was +++ for protein; the sediment contained 50 to 100 white cells and moderate numbers of tubular cells.

_____3. The patient had a habit of smoking one pack of cigarettes daily for 20 years but had stopped smoking for 30 years before admission.

_____4. On the patient's physical examination, there was no rash or lymphadenopathy, but petechiae were found.

_____5. The patient's urinary volume was 80 to 90 ml during each eight-hour shift on the second hospital day.

Answer the following questions according to the passage.

1. What symptoms did the patient have on the day of her admission?

_____

2. Do you think if there is any connection between the patient's history of smoking and drinking and her disease?

_____

3. Do you think when the patient can leave hospital?

_____

Use the appropriate form of the words or phrases in the box to complete the following sentences.

inflame	hematologic	ibuprofen	hydronephrosis	afebrile
endometrial	nebulizer	oliguria	skeletal	petechiae
moderate	diameter	electrocardiogram		

1. _____ toxicity now includes a statement to monitor blood counts and platelet counts during therapy with clofarabine intravenous injection.

2. As sick patients were hospitalized, the treatment given, usually a _____ that could clear clogged lung passages, could further disseminate virus.

3. Girls who begin menstruation earlier than the average have a greater chance of being short and fat and are at greater risk for breast cancer and _____ cancer later in life.

4. _____ (pinpoint hemorrhages) represents bleeding from small vessels and is classically found when a coagulopathy is present due to a low platelet count.

5. Many babies with _____ die before birth, because the diseased bladder retains urine that can severely damage the kidney.

6. To understand the clinical use of infrared ear the thermometer, 100_____ cases (oral temperature less than 37.5℃) were selected randomly as the control group.

7. If the child has unexplained crying, vomiting, fever, turbid urine, hematuria, urinary _____ even without the phenomenon requires an immediate visit to a local hospital.

8. Children who do not get enough vitamin D are at risk for rickets, a bone-softening disease that results in stunted growth and _____ deformities if not corrected while the child is young.

9. Baldwin said the girl has thrived in school and has no learning problems even though she has _____ asthma.

10. Chemical agents manufactured by our immune system _____ our

cells and tissues, causing our nose to run and our throat to swell.

Translation

A. Translate the following expressions into English.

1. 静脉给药
2. 阑尾切除术
3. 免疫球蛋白
4. 右外髂骨淋巴链
5. 低密度病灶
6. 轻微外周性水肿
7. 颈静脉压
8. 血液标本培养

B. Translate the following sentences or expressions into Chinese.

1. Ibuprofen and hydrochlorothiazide were discontinued, and intravenous administration of nonessential fluids was avoided.

2. She was advised to discontinue taking ibuprofen and to return for follow-up, but on the day of admission she vomited twice, felt extremely fatigued, continued to have malaise, and produced less urine than usual.

3. An abdominopelvic computed tomographic (CT) study revealed a small amount of pericardial thickening or fluid and minimal atelectasis at the base of the left lung.

4. She resided with her husband and had several children, one of whom had multiple sclerosis.

5. Two weeks later, malaise and a sensation of chilliness developed, with diffuse pains in the arms and legs, which prompted her to take two or three tablets of ibuprofen every four to five hours for two weeks.

Section C   Vocabulary (Terminology)

1. 肾 kidney

Combining Form	Meaning	Terminology	Terminology meaning
ren/o	kidney	renogram	a photographic depiction of the course of renal excretion of a radiolabeled substance 肾探测图
nephr/o	kidney	nephritis	acute or chronic inflammation of the kidney caused by infection, degenerative process, or vascular disease 肾炎

2. 肾盂 renal pelvis

Combining Form	Meaning	Terminology	Terminology meaning
pyel/o		pyelonephritis	inflammation of both the lining of the pelvis and the parenchyma of the kidney 肾盂肾炎

3. 肾盏 calix (calyx)

Combining Form	Meaning	Terminology	Terminology meaning
cali/o-	calyx or calix	caliectasis	肾盏扩张
calic/o		calyceal	肾盏的

4. 输尿管 ureter

Combining Form	Meaning	Terminology	Terminology meaning
ureter/o	ureter	ureteritis	inflammation of the ureters 输尿管炎

5. 膀胱 urinary bladder

Combining Form	Meaning	Terminology	Terminology meaning
cyst/o	urinary bladder	cystitis	inflammation of the urinary bladder 膀胱炎
vesci/o	urinary bladder	vesicoureteral reflux	膀胱输尿管返流

6. 尿道 urethra

Combining Form	Meaning	Terminology	Terminology meaning
urethra/o	urethra	urethritis	inflammation of the urethra 尿道炎
meat/o	meatus	meatal	of or relating to meatus 尿道的

7. 尿 urine, micturition

Combining Form	Meaning	Terminology	Terminology meaning
ur/o	urina(urea)	diuresis	an increased excretion of urine 利尿
urin/o	urine	urination	to discharge urine 排尿
-uria	urination	hematuria	the presence of blood or blood cells in the urine 血尿

8. 小球 glomerulus (collection of capillaries)

Combining Form	Meaning	Terminology	Terminology meaning
glomerul/o	glomerulus	glomerulonephritis	nephritis marked by inflammation of the capillaries of the renal glomeruli 肾小球肾炎

9. 白蛋白 albumin

Combining Form	Meaning	Terminology	Terminology meaning
albumin/o	albumin	albuminuria	the presence of albumin in the urine often symptomatic of kidney disease 蛋白尿

10. 氮 nitrogen

Combining Form	Meaning	Terminology	Terminology meaning
azot/o	nitrogen	azotemia	an excess of urea or other nitrogenous wastes in the blood as a result of kidney insufficiency 氮血症

11. 口渴 thirst

Combining Form	Meaning	Terminology	Terminology meaning
dips/o	thirst	polydipsia	excessive or abnormal thirst 烦渴

12. 酮体 ketone bodies

Combining Form	Meaning	Terminology	Terminology meaning
ket/o	ketone bodies (ketoacid and acetone)	ketosis	an abnormal increase of ketone bodies in the body 酮病
keton/o	Ketone bodies (ketoacids and acetone)	ketonuria	酮体尿

13. 夜晚 night

Combining Form	Meaning	Terminology	Terminology meaning
noct/i	night	nocturia	夜尿

14. 少 scanty

Combining Form	Meaning	Terminology	Terminology meaning
olig/o	scanty	oliguria	scanty in urine 少尿

15. 脓 pus

Combining Form	Meaning	Terminology	Terminology meaning
py/o	pus	pyuria	pus in the urine; *also*: a condition characterized by pus in the urine 脓尿

Exercise for vocabulary

Try to write down the meanings of the following terms that relate to urinary symptoms.

1. azotemia _____
2. polydipsia _____
3. oliguria _____
4. pyuria _____
5. albuminuria _____
6. urethritis _____
7. nephritis _____
8. hematuria _____
9. cystitis _____
10. glomerulonephritis _____

Match the following terms that pertain to urinalysis with their meanings below.

albuminuria	hematuria	phenylketonuria	sediment	bilirubinuria
ketonuria	pyuria	specific	gravity	glycosuria PH

_____1. Abnormal particles present in the urine cells. Bacteria, casts, and crystals

_____2. High levels of a substance appear in urine when a baby is born with a deficiency of an enzyme. The infant can become mentally retarded if she or he is not put on a strict diet that prevents the substance from accumulating in the blood and urine.

_____3. Smoky-red color of urine caused by the presence of blood.

_____4. Turbid(cloudy) urine caused by the presence of polymorphonuclear leukocytes and pus.

_____5. Sugar in the urine, a symptom of diabetes mellitus and a result of hyperglycemia.

_____6. This urine test reflects the acidity or alkalinity of the urine.

_____7. Dark pigment accumulates in urine as a result of liver or gallbladder diseases.

_____8. High levels of acids and acetones accumulate in the urine as a result of abnormal fat catabolism.

_____9. This urine test reflects the concentration of the urine.

_____10. Leaky glomeruli can produce accumulation of protein in the urine.

Fill in the blanks with the words given below.

nephrectomy	renal	hydronephrosis	calculi	nephrosclerosis
enuresis	hypotrophied	nephrologist		ketones
nephropathy				

1. After diagnosis of renal cell carcinoma (made by renal biopsy), Dr. John advised Alice that _____ would be necessary.

2. Ever since Bill's condition of gout was diagnosed, he has been warned that uric acid crystals could accumulate in his blood and tissues, leading to _____.

3. The voiding cystourethrogram demonstrated blockage of urine flow from Jim's bladder and _____.

4. Narrowed arterioles in the kidney increase blood pressure, and thus _____ ____ is often associated with hypertension.

5. Eight-year-old Willy continually wet his bed at night while sleeping. His mother

limited Willy's intake of fluids in the evening to discourage his _____.

6. Edmund's chronic juvenile diabetes eventually resulted in_____, which led to renal failure.

7. After Sue's bilateral renal failure, her doctor advised _____ to save her life.

8. When Betty's left kidney stopped functioning, her contralateral kidney overdeveloped or _____ to meet the increased workload.

9. A popular diet program recommends eating foods high in fats and protein. People on this diet check their urine for the presence of _____.

10. Andrea's urinalysis revealed proteinuria and her ankles began to swollen, demonstrating a condition known as edema, her _____ diagnosed Andrea's condition as nephrotic syndrome and recommended drugs to heal leaky glomeruli and diuretics to reduce swelling.

Section D   Writing

History of Past Illness (HPI)

在上一章讲了如何写主诉，我们在本章重点讲现病史（HPI）的写作。HPI 即使不是病历中最重要、最关键的部分，至少也是最重要、最关键的部分之一。HPI 是从医生角度，进一步描述主诉内容，全面说明现有疾病的起病时间与情况、主要症状的特点、疾病发展过程、症状间的关系、诊疗过程、目前患者的身体状况、与现有疾病有直接关系的过去情况等。HPI 也是反映医生全面采集了病史资料，在经思考之后，为阅读病历者合理地、有序地组织这些病史资料。因此，在书写病历之前，应该先把病例的各个方面从头到尾思考一遍，再组织病历资料。

HPI 是对现有相关病史资料和既往原始数据深思熟虑后（通常按照时间先后顺序）有序的编辑总结，它使读者通过患者的临床表现作出鉴别诊断，得出与在病史最后作出的初步诊断一致的诊断或一组诊断。书写 HPI 时应该使用完整的语句，至于时态，记述患者入院情况多用一般过去时或过去完成时，而叙述目前病情时一般用一般现在时或现在完成时。完整的 HPI 包括以下四部分：

1. 对原始主诉或需要强调的事件的陈述。

2. 与那些一路领先相关的背景资料，包括那些与你关注的临床表现相关的以前曾获得的原始资料、伴随症状、社会状况、个人习惯或暴露史。

3. 对主诉特点的解释（例如病程时间、放射性状、加重因素）。

4. 有助于鉴别诊断的相关阳性症状和阴性症状。

以下是一个完整的 HPI 的例子：

Example 1: M.T. is a 45-year-old homeless Vietnamese male who was in his usual state of health until approximately 5 weeks prior to admission when he began noting drenching night sweats occurring initially about 2 times weekly (Chief complaint). The night sweats then increased in frequency, and about 3 weeks prior to admission, he also began having a cough. It was initially dry but progressed to being productive of small amounts yellow sputum tinged with blood. He also thinks he had fevers but had no access to thermometer. He has been staying at various shelters around Boston. He noted that he'd been losing about 5 lbs/month without trying to diet and there had been no change in his activity level. This had been going on for about 3 months. He had no history of injection drug use, blood transfusion, or cigarette use and does not know his PPD status. He has had multiple sexual partners over the last few years when he has been on the streets, including 2 experiences of trading unprotected sex with another male for alcohol. The patient admits to only sporadic condom use and says he forgets when he gets drunk, which happens a few times a week. He had an uncomplicated admission in 2/97 to St. Else for community-acquired pneumonia. He stated that there were a lot of people at the shelters who had "cold" but didn't know any specifics about those illness. M.T. came to the USA about 10 years ago and has lived in Boston the entire time with no travel outside the city. At this time, he denies dyspnea, chest pain, nausea, vomiting, diarrhea, swollen lymph node, myalgias, arthralgias, decreased appetite and rash.

Exercise

Write the following history of past illness.

1. 现病史：患者 3 年来于秋冬季节反复发作上腹剑突下饥饿样隐痛不适，多于空腹发作，餐后 2～3 小时或后半夜发生，进食后有所减轻，时有反酸、嗳气。曾间断服用"雷尼替丁"，腹痛能控制。昨天下午 4 时又发剑突下腹痛，呈持续性、烧灼样疼痛，程度较以往重，服用"654-2"不能缓解。下午 6 时有便意，后解柏油样、稀糊状黑便 4 次，总量约为 1000mL，便后腹痛缓解，但患者自觉乏力、头昏、心悸、口干。病程中无食欲减退、进行性消瘦、吞咽困难、无恶心、呕吐、黄疸、发热、无呕血、鲜血便。为进一步诊治收住院。患者精神差，睡眠欠佳，近 8 小时尿量约 400mL，已 4 小时未解大便。

2. 现病史：患者有 4 年糖尿病史，进行饮食控制，情况一直很好，直到半年前，开始感到较前虚弱。两个月前她接受眼睑手术时，发现血糖偏高，予甲糖宁（甲苯磺丁脲）500mg，每日 3 次。入院前 2～3 天，患有上呼吸道感染，患者家属说病情加重，社区医院给予抗生素治疗，烦躁不安两天，食欲不振。咳黄痰，尿糖+++，但酮体阴性。今晨发现焦急不安，神志不清，沉默寡语。

Section E   Spoken English

Role play

Directions: A patient got kidney stones, on and off for about 3 months with a severe bout of pain in his back, he went to clinic for help. 2 students are selected to demonstrate the conversation, one plays the role of doctor, the other plays the role of patient.

Discussion

Directions: Work in groups and discuss with your partners, then answer the following questions with detailed analysis.

A 22-year-old female presents to the ED with 3 days of increased urinary frequency and suprapubic pain after micturition. She has no fever, chill, or flank pain, nausea or vomiting, and urethral discharge. There have been no similar complaints in the past. She is sexually active and uses a barrier mode of contraception. She has no history of sexually transmitted diseases. She has no allergy to medications or food. Physical examination is unremarkable. Spot urinary pregnancy test is negative. Urinalysis is significant for 12 white blood cells (WBCs) and 3 red blood cells (RBCs), and the urine is nitrite positive. She has no primary care physician.

What is the diagnosis and the next step of action?

Terminology related to kidney and urine department

acute renal failure 急性肾功能衰竭

chronic renal failure 慢性肾功能衰竭

blood purification 血液净化

peritoneal dialysis 腹膜透析

intermittent peritoneal dialysis 间歇性腹膜透析

continuous peritoneal dialysis 连续性腹膜透析

plasma exchange 血浆置换

primary glomerular diseases 原发性肾小球疾病

acute glomerulonephritis 急性肾小球肾炎

acute rapidly progressive glomerulonephritis 急进性肾小球肾炎

chronic glomerulonephritis 慢性肾小球肾炎

nephrotic syndrome 肾病综合征

renal replacement 肾移植

minimal change nephropathy 微小病变肾病

IgA nephropathy IgA 肾病

urinary tract infection 泌尿道感染

pyelonephritis 肾盂肾炎

cystitis 膀胱炎

acute urethral syndrome 急性尿道综合征

interstitial nephritis 间质性肾炎

renal papillary necrosis 肾乳头坏死

renal tubular acidosis 肾小管酸中毒

obstructive nephropathy 梗阻性肾病

renal calculi 肾石病

nephrolithiasis 肾石病

cystic disease of the kidney 肾脏囊肿性疾病

simple renal cystic disease 单纯性肾囊肿

polycystic kidney disease 多囊肾

urinalysis 尿分析

renal cell carcinoma(hypernephroma) 肾上腺样瘤

renal hypertension 肾性高血压

bladder cancer 膀胱癌

blood urea nitrogen 血尿素氮

endogenous creatinine clearance test 内生肌酐清除率

glomerular filtration rate 肾小球滤过率

serum creatinine 血清肌酐

urine volume 尿量

hemoglobinuria 血红蛋白尿

bilirubinuira 胆红素尿

pyuria 脓尿

bacteriuria 菌尿

chyluria 乳糜尿

lipiduria 脂肪尿

hematochyluria 乳糜血尿

proteinuria 蛋白尿

pathological proteinuria 病理性蛋白尿

glomerular proteinuria 肾小球性蛋白尿

tubular proteinuria 肾小管性蛋白尿

mixed proteinuria 混合性蛋白尿

overflow proteinuria 溢出性蛋白尿

false proteinuria 假性蛋白尿

ketone bodies　酮体

ketonuria　酮尿

urobilinogen　尿胆原

urine amylase　尿淀粉酶

CT scan　CT 扫描

intravenous pyelogram　静脉肾盂造影

renal angiography　肾血管造影

retrograde pyelogram　逆行肾盂造影

retrograde urethrography　逆行尿道造影

cystoscopy　膀胱镜检查

renal biopsy　肾活检

renal transplantation　肾移植

urinary catheterization　尿导管插入术

Useful expressions in writing documents

1. 起病的性质和特征

begin explosively　爆发性发病

fulminating/ explosive　爆发性的

gradual　缓慢的

emergency　急症

abrupt attack/sudden onset/attack began all of sudden　突然发作

occurred rapidly　迅速出现

2. 症状所在的部位

anterior　前面的，前部的，以前的；较早的

at the left part of …　在左侧的

in the left lumbar region　在左侧背部

in the right upper quadrant of …　在右上腹部

in the right side of …　在右侧

posterior　后面的；尾部的；背部的，较晚的，以后的

subcutaneous　皮下的

subphrenic　膈下的

3. 症状的性质、特征、程度

focal　病灶的

afebrile　不发热的

unbearable　不可忍受的

continuous/persistent　持续的

paroxysmal　阵发性的

acute 急性的

spastic 痉挛的

local 局部的

bearable 可忍受的

palpable 可以触及的

chronic 慢性的

apparent/clear/obvious/definite/distinct 明显的

septic 败血症的

prodromal symptom 前驱症状

mild 轻度的

constitutional/general/generalized/systemic 全身性的

asymptomatic 无症状的

severe 严重的

moderate 中等程度的

4. 出现的频率

recurrent/variable 反复不定的

relapsing 复发的

intermittent 间歇性的

frequent 频繁的

transient 一过性的

5. 各种症状的关系

concomitant symptom 伴随症状

be accompanied by/associated with 伴有

primary 原发的

secondary 继发的

precipitating 诱发的

follow 接着

precede 先行，先于

6. 病情的发展

persist

be more severe/worsen

have a relapse/recur

improve

be better/improving

be relieved

aggravate/be exacerbated

subside

decline

recover

disappear

heal

（1）症状好转

feel better than before

take a favorable turn

take a turn for the better

improve

make favorable progress

turn for the better

change for the better

be better

（2）症状减轻

alleviate

reduce

palliate

diminish

ease(lighten)

mitigate

（3）症状消失

disappear

subside

regress

clear up

vanish

dissolve

die (fade) away

relieve

（4）症状加重

be (make, become, get) worse

worsen

become more severe

take a turn for the worse

be aggravated

increase in severity

take a bad turn

make (become) more serious

make (become) heavier

（5）无变化

remain the same as......

continue without change

be identical

be alike

be similar

resemble

（6）时好时坏

wane and wax

hang in the balance

7. 治疗经过

had...... previous hospitalizations

saw his/her family doctor

was treated by the local physician

was referred to the hospital

was admitted for work-up

was treated symptomatically

started on medicine

remained the same/was unchanged

Chapter 6

Nervous System

Section A   Focus Listening

Conversation

Listen to the dialogue and fill in the blanks with proper words.

P=patient D=doctor

P: Doctor, I'm having a bad headache.

D: How long have you had this pain?

P: Since yesterday.

D: Is this the first episode?

P: Yes, it is.

D: Which part of your head is affected? Can you show me exactly where the pain is?

P: Here, it is just on the right side of my head.

D: What kind of pain is it?

P: It felt like a _____ pain.

D: Does it come suddenly?

P: No, I am depressed, restless and nervous because I didn't do well in my registered accountant test a week ago.

D: Did you experience any other discomfort?

P: Yes, I experienced light _____, blurred vision, sound sensitivity, irritability, malaise, loss of appetite and thirst.

D: Any other symptoms following?

P: Yeah, some visual alteration, hemianopic field defects, scotoma and scintillation, and the most frightening was that I felt numb in my right face.

D: Is the pain persistent or intermittent, can you describe it?

P: Intermittent and throbbing which lasted about 16 hours, but sometime it seems boring and can radiate to the opposite of head.

D: Does anything special make it worse?

P: Yes, it's aggravated on exertion or by shaking my head.

D: Does anything relieve it?

P: Yes, it can be abated after sleeping.

D: You are highly suspected to suffer from the _____ with aura, which is manifested by headache that is usually unilateral and frequently pulsatile in quality, it often associated with nausea, vomiting, photophobia (light sensitivity), phonophobia (sound sensitivity) and lassitude. I'll prescribe some medications to kill the pain.

About an hour later, the patient came in the doctor's office for further _____.

P: Doctor, you know, the pain is severe. Can it be cured?

D: Not yet, the therapy is only to alleviate the pain or terminate the bout of migraine and prevent the recurrence.

P: Does the migraine often recur?

D: It depends. If the migraine attacks you over 3 times a month, you should come here to accept _____ therapy.

P: Does anything precipitate the occurrence of migraine?

D: Yes, for example, certain food, such as cheese, meat, hot dog and bacon which contain tyramine, emotion, menses drug such as nitroglycerin and bright lights may also trigger the attacks.

New Words & Expressions

throb 跳动，悸动

malaise 不安

hemianopia 偏盲

scotoma 暗点

scintillation 闪光

photophobia 畏光，恐光症

phonophobia 畏声

lassitude 无力，没精打采

migraine 偏头痛

tyramine 酪胺

trigger 触发

Passage

Answer the questions after listening to the passage.

1. Cerebral palsy is most commonly manifested in_____.

A. new born babies

B. adults

C. children

D. old age

2. What are the types of CP?

A. Spastic cerebral palsy.   B. Dyskinetic cerebral palsy.

C. Ataxic cerebral palsy.   D. All of the above.

3. Which one of the following is common in CP?

A. Loss of motor function.   B. Loss of sensory function.

C. Loss of muscles.   D. Both A and B.

4. Which one of the following is NOT a symptom of CP?

A. Loss of balance.   B. Loss of vision.

C. Difficulty in breathing.   D. Loss of blood.

5. Which one of the following conditions is result of CP?

A. Vision loss.   B. Hearing loss.

C. Inability to learn.   D. All of the above.

Section B　Reading Comprehension

Text

A 57-year-old right-handed man was admitted to the hospital because of the sudden onset of slurred speech and left hemiparesis. The patient had been well until two days earlier, when he fell and fractured his left humerus. His daily aspirin was discontinued because of the fracture. At 2 p.m. he was last seen well by his mother-in-law who noted that he was drooling at 2:15 p.m., had slurred speech, and could not swallow pills. She called his wife, who came home from work immediately and found him unable to move his left arm or leg. He stated that he did not have a headache, nausea, or neck pain. He was brought to the hospital by ambulance at 4:30 p.m.

The patient had a history of coronary and bilateral carotid-artery atherosclerosis. Combined coronary-artery bypass grafting and left internal carotid endarterectomy had been performed for 16 months before admission. He had asymptomatic, mild-to-moderate stenosis of the right internal carotid artery, well-controlled hypertension, hyperlipidemia, degenerative arthritis, and borderline diabetes and was obese. His medications were fluvastatin, irbesartan, ibuprofen, aspirin, and acetaminophen with oxycodone as needed for the recent fracture. He was allergic to penicillin. He lived with his wife and was employed as a civil servant. He had smoked and consumed alcohol in moderation in the past but had stopped doing both at the time of coronary-artery bypass grafting. There was no history of atrial fibrillation, clotting disorders, cardiac valvular disease, or use of illicit drugs. The temperature was 36 ℃ , the pulse 94 beats per minute, and the respirations

20 breaths per minute. The blood pressure was 178/84 mmHg. The oxygen saturation was greater than 98 percent while the patient was breathing ambient air. On physical examination, he appeared acutely ill. The neck was supple and non-tender. The carotid pulses were equal, and there were no bruits. The lungs were clear, and he could lie flat without aspiration or respiratory difficulty. The heart sounds were normal. The limbs were well perfused, and the abdomen was normal.

On neurologic examination, he was alert and oriented, and although he was inattentive, he was able to recall recent events. He exhibited dense neglect (lack of awareness) with respect to objects or stimuli on his left side. He was unaware of his own deficits (a state termed anosognosia) and thought he was in the hospital for his heart condition. His left arm was in a sling when it was held in front of him and he identified it as belonging to the examiner. He had mild dysarthria, but his speech was fluent and his comprehension, repetition, and naming abilities were intact.

He had complete left-sided homonymous hemianopia. The optic disks and retinal vessels were normal, the pupils were equal and reactive, and there was no ptosis. There was a conjugate rightward gaze deviation; he could not direct his gaze voluntarily past midline or to the left. On his left face, he had severe weakness and no sensation of a pin prick. The head turned to the right. The tongue was midline and moved well.

There was normal tone and full strength in the right arm and leg. He could not make voluntary movements with his left arm and leg, although occasionally the left leg spontaneously stiffened in extension. The deep tendon reflexes were normal on the right side and absent on the left. Plantar stimulation produced plantar flexion on the right and triple flexion (flexion of the hip and knee and dorsiflexion of the ankle) on the left. Gait testing was deferred. His score on the National Institutes of Health Stroke Scale (NIHSS) (which ranges from 0 to 34, with higher scores indicating greater deficits) was 20. The results of urinalysis included 3+ glucose but were otherwise normal. Other laboratory values are shown in figure 3.

Table 1. Laboratory Values on Admission.*	
Variable	Value
Sodium (mmol/liter)	137
Blood urea nitrogen (mg/dl)	11
Creatinine (mg/dl)	0.8
Glucose (mg/dl)	270
White cells (per mm³)	12,300
Hematocrit (%)	39.6
Platelets (per mm³)	232,000
Prothrombin time (sec)	12.8†
Activated partial-thromboplastin time (sec)	21.4
Calcium (mg/dl)	7.1
Magnesium (mmol/liter)	0.65
Creatine kinase (U/liter)	201
Creatine kinase isoenzyme (ng/ml)	1.3
Troponin T (ng/ml)	<0.01
Albumin (g/dl)	2.1
Cholesterol (mg/dl)	
Total	147
High-density lipoprotein	37
Low-density lipoprotein	88
Triglyceride (mg/dl)	112
Functional protein S (% of normal value)	71
Functional protein C (% of normal value)	79
Anticardiolipin antibody‡	
IgG (GPL units)	2.2
IgM (MPL units)	1.8
Lupus anticoagulant	Negative
Activated protein C resistance	2.6

* To convert the value for blood urea nitrogen to millimoles per liter, multiply by 0.357. To convert the value for creatinine to micromoles per liter, multiply by 88.4. To convert the value for glucose to millimoles per liter, multiply by 0.05551. To convert the value for calcium to millimoles per liter, multiply by 0.250. To convert the value for magnesium to milliequivalents per liter, divide by 0.5. To convert the values for cholesterol to millimoles per liter, multiply by 0.02586. To convert the value for triglyceride to millimoles per liter, multiply by 0.01129.
† The control value was 12.3 seconds.
‡ GPL denotes IgG phospholipid, and MPL IgM phospholipid.

Figure 3 Table of laboratory values

An electrocardiogram showed a sinus rhythm at a rate of 94 beats per minute with minor, nonspecific ST-segment and T-wave abnormalities. Chest radiographs showed evidence of a previous median sternotomy, clear lungs, and a normal cardiomediastinal silhouette. A cardiac ultrasonographic examination showed no vegetations, intracardiac thrombus, segmental wall-motion abnormalities, intracardiac shunts, or valvular disease.

Dr. James D. Rabinov: A computed tomographic (CT) scan of the head, obtained without the use of contrast material, shows a dense right middle cerebral artery, calcification of the basal ganglia on the left side, and no evidence of acute intracranial hemorrhage (Figure 4).

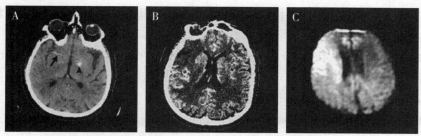

Figure 4 Images of the brain on admission

Subtle hypoattenuation is seen in the right insular region, lentiform nuclei, and frontal lobe, with effacement of the sulci in the right frontal lobe.

A cranial CT scan, obtained without the use of contrast material (Panel A), shows a dense right middle cerebral artery (arrow), indicating the presence of a clot in the vessel. Benign calcifications are present in the basal ganglia on the left side (arrowhead). A perfusion window of the axial image of the CT angiogram (Panel B) shows hypoperfusion in the right frontal operculum, manifested as a dark area within the cortex. A diffusion-weighted MRI scan (Panel C) shows that diffusion is restricted (bright area) in the right frontal lobe, indicating the presence of acute infarction.

New Words & Expressions

hemiparesis [hemɪpəˈriːsɪs] *n.* 轻偏瘫，偏身轻瘫

fracture [ˈfræktʃə] *v.* break (a bone) 使破裂，折断

coronary [ˈkɔrənɛri] *a.* relating to the heart 冠状动脉的；心脏的，与心脏有关的

atherosclerosis [ˌæθərəʊsklɪˈrəʊsɪs] *n.* a stage of arteriosclerosis involving fatty deposits inside the arterial walls 动脉粥样硬化；动脉硬化

carotid [kəˈrɑtɪd] *a.* of or relating to either of the two major arteries supplying blood to the head and neck 颈动脉的

endarterectomy [ˌɛndɑrtəˈrektəmi] *n.* 动脉内膜切除术

asymptomatic [ˌesɪmptəˈmætɪk] *a.* having no symptoms of illness or disease 无症状的

illicit [ɪˈlɪsɪt] *a.* contrary to or forbidden by law 违法的；不正当的

stimuli [ˈstɪmjʊlaɪ] *n.* any stimulating information or event 刺激；刺激物

dysarthria[dɪsˈɑːθrɪə] *n.* impaired articulatory ability resulting from defects in the peripheral motor nerves or in the speech musculature 构音障碍；构音困难

homonymous [hɒˈmɒnɪməs] *a.* of or related to or being homonyms 同名的；双关的

hemianopia [ˌhemɪənˈəʊpɪə] *n.* blindness in one half of the visual field of one or both eyes 偏盲；一侧视力缺失

conjugate [ˈkɒndʒəgeɪt] *a.* joined together especially in a pair or pairs 共轭的；结合的

plantar [ˈplæntə] *a.* relating to or occurring on the undersurface of the foot [解剖]跖的；脚底的

sternotomy [stəˈnɒtəmi] *n.* 胸骨切开术

lentiform [ˈlentifɔːm] *a.* convex on both sides; shaped like a lentil 透镜的；小扁豆似的

lentil [ˈlentl] *n.* round flat seed of the lentil plant used for food 兵豆，小扁豆

operculum [əʊˈpɜːkjʊləm] *n.* [昆]盖；鳃盖

Exercise

Decide whether the following statements are true (T) or false (F) according to the passage.

_____1. The patient had been well until two days earlier, when he fell and fractured his right humerus.

_____2. He had smoked and consumed alcohol in moderation in the past but had stopped doing both at the time of coronary-artery bypass grafting.

_____3. The patient was alert and oriented during neurologic examination, and he was able to recall recent events even though he was inattentive.

_____4. The patient had a little slight weakness and no sensation of a pin prick in his left face.

_____5. The patient's cardiac ultrasonographic examination showed some vegetations, intracardiac thrombus, segmental wall-motion abnormalities, intracardiac shunts, or valvular disease.

Answer the following questions according to the passage.

1. What is your diagnosis based on the figures?

_____

2. What medication should you pay attention to when you prescribe since the patient was allergic to penicillin?

_____

3. What advice will you give when the patient is discharge from hospital?

_____

Use the appropriate form of the words or phrases in the box to complete the following sentences.

plantar	acetaminophen	sternotomy	hemiparesis	
coronary	hemianopia	conjugate	asymptomatic	
carotid	illicit	fracture	stimuli	nontender

1. When a bone is broken in more than two places or gets crushed, the name for it is a comminuted _____.

2. This beating-heart technique avoids _____, cardiopulmonary bypass, and aortic cross-clamping but carries specific intra-operative anesthetic concerns and complications.

3. According to the American Heart Association (AHA), at least half of the people who die suddenly from _____ heart disease each year had no clue they were sick.

4. Unfortunately, often the arms and manpower fueling these conflicts are tied to transnational criminal activity through _____ trade in drugs, diamonds, and people.

5. All identified close contacts including the other members of the affected family and involved health care workers remain _____ and have been removed from close medical observation.

6. To check your pulse over your _____ artery, place your index and middle fingers on your neck to the side of your windpipe.

7. The patients had chronic _____, which is weakness on one side of the body, at least six months after a stroke.

8. HSN is a right cerebral hemisphere disease relating to cognitive impairment while homonymous _____ is the defect of visual field.

9. A second reason for persistence is that the activity itself creates _____ that _____ focus attention towards its continuance and completion.

10. This is a great exercise to "wake up" the deep muscles within the foot that help support the arch and _____ fascia ligament.

Translation

A. Translate the following expressions into English.

1. 口齿不清
2. 急性颅内出血
3. 左颈内动脉内膜切除术
4. 步态检查
5. 退行性关节炎
6. 心房颤动
7. 视网膜血管
8. 同向偏盲

B. Translate the following sentences or expressions into Chinese.

1. At 2 p.m. he was last seen well by his mother-in-law who noted that he was drooling at 2:15 p.m., had slurred speech, and could not swallow pills.

2. He was unaware of his own deficits (a state termed anosognosia) and thought he was in the hospital for his heart condition.

3. There was a conjugate rightward gaze deviation; he could not direct his gaze voluntarily past midline or to the left.

4. He could not make voluntary movements with his left arm and leg, although occasionally the left leg spontaneously stiffened in extension.

5. An electrocardiogram showed a sinus rhythm at a rate of 94 beats per minute with minor, nonspecific ST-segment, and T-wave abnormalities.

Section C　Vocabulary (Terminology)

1. 脑 brain, encephalon

Combining form	Meaning	Terminology	Terminology meaning
encephal/o	brain	encephalitis	inflammation of the brain 脑炎

2. 大脑 cerebrum

Combining form	Meaning	Terminology	Terminology meaning
cerebr/o	cerebrum	cerebrovascular	of or involving the cerebrum and the blood vessels supplying it 脑血管的

3. 小脑 cerebellum

Combining form	Meaning	Terminology	Terminology meaning
cerebell/o	cerebellum	cerebellar	of or involving the cerebellum 小脑的

4. 丘脑 thalamus

Combining form	Meaning	Terminology	Terminology meaning
thalam/o	thalamus	thalamic	of or involving the thalamus 丘脑的

5. 脑桥 pons

Combining form	Meaning	Terminology	Terminology meaning
pont/o	pons	cerebellopontine	of or involving the cerebellum and pons 小脑脑桥的

6. 皮质 cortex

Combining form	Meaning	Terminology	Terminology meaning
cortic/o	cortex	corticosteroid	any of various adrenal-cortex steroids (as corticosterone, cortisone, and aldosterone) used medically especially as anti-inflammatory agents 皮质类固醇

7. 硬膜 dura mater

Combining form	Meaning	Terminology	Terminology meaning
dur/o	dura mater	epidural	situated upon or administered or placed outside the dura mater 硬膜上的

8. 胶质 glue

Combining form	Meaning	Terminology	Terminology meaning
gli/o	glue, parts of the nervous system that support and connect	glioblastoma	a malignant rapidly growing astrocytoma of the central nervous system and usually of a cerebral hemisphere 成胶质细胞瘤

9. 脑膜 meninges

Combining form	Meaning	Terminology	Terminology meaning
mening/o	membranes, meninges	meningitis	inflammation of the meninges and especially of the pia mater and the arachnoid 脑膜炎
meningi/o	membranes, meninges	meningioma	a slow-growing encapsulated typically benign tumor arising from the meninges and often causing damage by pressing upon the brain and adjacent parts 脑膜瘤

10. 神经 nerve

Combining form	Meaning	Terminology	Terminology meaning
neur/o	nerve	neuropathy	an abnormal and usually degenerative state of the nervous system or nerves; *also*: a systemic condition that stems from a neuropathy 神经病

11. 神经根 nerve root

Combining form	Meaning	Terminology	Terminology meaning
radicul/o	nerve root	radiculitis	an inflammation of the nerve root 神经根炎

12. 鞘 sheath

Combining form	Meaning	Terminology	Terminology meaning
thec/o	sheath	intrathecal	introduced into or occurring in the space under the arachnoid membrane of the brain or spinal cord 鞘内的

14. 迷走神经 vagus

Combining form	Meaning	Terminology	Terminology meaning
vag/o	vagus	vagotomy	surgical division of the vagus nerve 迷走神经切断术

15. 交感神经 sympathetic nerve

Combining form	Meaning	Terminology	Terminology meaning
sympathy/o	sympathetic nerve	sympathoblast	成交感神经细胞

16. 骨髓 bone marrow, medulla

Combining form	Meaning	Terminology	Terminology meaning
myel/o	bone marrow	myeloblast	a large mononuclear nongranular bone-marrow cell; *especially*: one that is a precursor of a myelocyte 成髓细胞
		Myeloma	a primary tumor of the bone marrow 骨髓瘤

17. 疼痛 pain

Combining form	Meaning	Terminology	Terminology meaning
-algia	pain	neuralgia	acute paroxysmal pain radiating along the course of one or more nerves usually without demonstrable changes in the nerve structure 神经痛
-dynia	pain	pleurodynia	胸膜痛

18. 痛觉过敏 excessive sensitivity to pain

Combining form	Meaning	Terminology	Terminology meaning
alges/o	excessive sensitivity to pain	analgesia	insensibility to pain without loss of consciousness 痛觉缺失
-algesia		hypalgesia	痛觉减退

19. 感觉 feeling, nervous sensation

Combining form	Meaning	Terminology	Terminology meaning
esthesi/o	feeling, nervous sensation	anesthesia	loss of sensation with or without loss of consciousness 麻醉
-esthesia		hyperesthesia	unusual or pathological sensitivity of the skin or of a particular sense 感觉过敏

20. 烧灼感 burning

Combining form	Meaning	Terminology	Terminology meaning
caus/o	burning	causalgia	a constant usually burning pain resulting from injury to a peripheral nerve 灼痛

21. 运动 movement

Combining form	Meaning	Terminology	Terminology meaning
kines/o		bradykinesia	运动过慢，身心反应迟钝
-kinesis	movement	hyperkinesis	abnormally increased and sometimes uncontrollable activity or muscular movements
-kinetic		akinetic	运动不能的

22. 疾病发作 seizure

Combining form	Meaning	Terminology	Terminology meaning
-lepsy	seizure	epilepsy	any of various disorders marked by abnormal electrical discharges in the brain and typically manifested by sudden brief episodes of altered or diminished consciousness, involuntary movements, or convulsions 癫痫；羊痫风

23. 轻瘫 slight paralysis

Combining form	Meaning	Terminology	Terminology meaning
-paresis	slight paralysis	hemiparesis	slight paralysis of half body 轻偏瘫

24. 言语 speech

Combining form	Meaning	Terminology	Terminology meaning
-phasis	speech	aphasias	loss or impairment of the power to use or comprehend words usually resulting from brain damage 失语症

25. 瘫痪 paralysis(loss or impairment of the ability to move parts of the body)

Combining form	Meaning	Terminology	Terminology meaning
-plegia	paralysis	hemiplegia	total or partial paralysis of one side of the body that results from disease of or injury to the motor centers of the brain 偏瘫

26. 动作 action

Combining form	Meaning	Terminology	Terminology meaning
-praxia	action	apraxia	loss or impairment of the ability to execute complex coordinated movements without muscular or sensory impairment 失用

27. 力量 strength

Combining form	Meaning	Terminology	Terminology meaning
-sthenia	strength	neurasthenia	a psychological disorder marked especially by easy fatigability and often by lack of motivation, feelings of inadequacy, and psychosomatic symptoms 神经衰弱

28. 死亡 to cut off , cut short

Combining form	Meaning	Terminology	Terminology meaning
syncope/o	to cut off , cut short	syncope	loss of consciousness resulting from insufficient blood flow to the brain 晕厥

Exercise for vocabulary

Try to write down the meanings of the following terms related to nervous symptoms.

1. astrocytoma _____

2. pyogenic meningitis _____

3. cerebral contusion _____

4. cerebrovascular accident _____

5. cerebral thrombosis _____

6. HIV encephalopathy _____

7. hypalgesia _____

8. motor aphasia _____

9. comatose _____

10. paresthesia _____

Match the following terms pertaining to urinalysis with their meanings below.

migraine	contusion and subdural	hematoma	glioblastoma	TIA
myasthenia	gravis meningitis	dyslexia	hemiparesis	
syncopal	Alzheimer disease			

1. Suzy had such severe headaches that she could find relief only with strong analgesics. Her condition of _____ was debilitating.

2. Frederico was in a coma after his high-speed car accident. His physicians were concerned that he had suffered a _____ as a result of the accident.

3. Dick went to the emergency department complaining of dizziness, nausea, and headache. The physician, suspecting ICP, prescribed corticosteroids, and Dick's symptoms disappeared. They returned, however, when the steroid was discontinued. A (an) revealed a large brain lesion. It was removed surgically and determined to be a(n) _____.

4. Dorothy felt tingling sensations in her hand and noticed blurred vision and numbness in her arm, all signs of _____. Her physician requested MRA to assess any damage to cerebral blood vessels and possible stroke.

5. When Bill noticed muscle weakness in his face, he reported these symptoms to his doctor. The doctor diagnosed his condition as _____ and prescribed anticholinesterase drugs, which relieved his symptoms.

6. To rule out bacterial _____, Dr. Phillips, a pediatrician, requested a LP be performed on the febrile (feverish) child.

7. Seven-year-old Barry reversed his letters and had difficulty learning to read and write words. His family physician diagnosed his problem as _____.

8. After his head hit the steering wheel during a recent automobile accident, Clark noticed _____ on the left side of his body. A head CT scan revealed.

9. For her 35th birthday, Elizabeth's husband threw her a surprise party. She was so startled by the crowd that she experienced a weakness of muscles and loss of consciousness. Friends placed her on her back in a horizontal position with her head low to improve blood flow to her brain. she soon recovered from her _____ episode.

10. Near her 65th birthday, Estelle began having difficulty in recent events. Over the next five years, she developed age-related dementia and was diagnosed _____.

Section D   Writing

Past Medical History (PMH)

在既往史中，一要详尽列举既往疾病和事件，二要列举包括支持资料（比如可得到的活检资料、肺功能检查、超声、X线、CT等），三要分述手术史、妊娠生育史和精神病史。但也有人将既往病史与手术史、精神病史、妊娠生育史分开叙述，这可以根据你所在医疗机构以及你自己的习惯而定。在整理既往史时，对于有具体发生时间的事件（如个体检查、某个事件，如一次卒中或一次手术），须按时间顺序罗列，对于一些慢性疾病（如糖尿病或慢性阻塞性肺气肿）的诊断，可按疾病的严重程度或疾病的活动程度罗列。既往史是记录患者过去患病与治疗情况，谓语动词常用一般过去时、过去完成时，偶尔用过去进行时。

Example:

1. Congestive heart failure. Last ultrasound in April 2001: moderate left ventricular hypertrophy, left ventricular ejection fraction = 35%, moderate left atrioventricular valve regurgitation/right atrioventricular valve regurgitation. In August 1998, the New York Heart Function Class Ⅱ was diagnosed by Dr. Ven Trikel of the Heart Failure Division.

2. Type Ⅱ diabetes. Diagnosed in 1993 with mild retinopathy (last ophthalmological examination in September 1998) and toe neuropathy. The last urine microprotein assay was negative in February 2003. Self-testing of blood sugar was conducted 3 times a week, the last glycated hemoglobin value in January 2009 was 8.1.

3. Cholecystectomy due to gallstones was performed in April 1994.

4. Hypertension. well controlled for the past 5 years.

5. Hysterectomy was possibly performed at Boston Hospital in 1990, with details unknown.

1. 充血性心力衰竭。2001 年 4 月末次超声检查：中度左心室肥厚，左室射血分数为 35%，中度左房室瓣回流 / 右房室瓣回流。1998 年 8 月纽约心功能分级Ⅱ级，由心衰门诊的 Ven Trikel 医师诊断。

2. 2 型糖尿病。1993 年确诊，并发轻度视网膜病变（最后一次眼科检查是 1998 年 9 月）和足趾神经病变。2003 年 2 月最后一次尿微量蛋白测定阴性。每周 3 次自测血糖，2009 年 1 月最后一次糖化血红蛋白值为 8.1。

3. 1994 年 4 月因胆结石行胆囊切除术。

4. 高血压。近 5 年血压控制满意。

5. 可能于 1990 年在波士顿行子宫切除术，具体不详。

Exercise

Write the following MPH.

1. HIV+，1997 年 5 月确诊，应用抗逆转录病毒药物三联治疗 18 个月，2002 年 11 月，2002 年 11 月末次 CD4 检测为 320，HIV 病毒负荷不详。合并有鹅口疮，1998 年 4 月曾患卡氏肺孢子虫肺炎。

2. 1995 年曾诊断为三尖瓣性心内膜炎，草绿色链球菌感染，原因为静脉注射海洛因。1997 年 1 月超声：轻度三尖瓣反流，其余指标均在正常范围内。

3. 静脉药物应用：以前用海洛因，现用美沙酮维持。

4. 左大腿黑色素瘤，1998 年确诊。病理：浅表扩散，深度为 0.62mm。在波士顿医学中心行切除术，边缘距病灶 2cm，术后无复发。

5. PPD+。1997 年采用异烟肼治疗 6 个月。

6. 十余岁时患水痘，并发肺炎。

7. 孕 3 产 2，自然流产 1 次。

Section E   Spoken English

Role play

Directions: A patient complained of intermittent dizziness and weakness of limbs for over 5 years, he went to clinic for help. 5 students are selected to demonstrate the conversation. Four play the role of Dr. Liu, Dr. Zhu, Dr. Xiao, Dr. Zhao, the last one plays the role of patient.

Discussion

Directions: Work in groups and discuss with your partners, then answer the following questions with detailed analysis.

Mrs. Oswald is a 78-year-old female who presents to the emergency department with a 2-hour history of slurred speech. She also complains of difficulty with word-finding and right-sided weakness and numbness. She denies any vision changes, headache, fever, trauma, chest pain, or abdominal pain. She has a history of hypertension, hyperlipidemia, and atrial fibrillation. Her medications include hydrochlorothiazide, metoprolol, fish oil, and aspirin. She has not taken warfarin for the last 3 years after an incident of diverticular bleeding. She does not smoke or use alcohol. On examination, she is awake yet anxious, with a blood pressure of 194/102 mmHg, heart rate of 116 bpm, respiratory rate of 20 breaths/min, and oxygen saturation of 96% on room air. Chest auscultation reveals clear lungs and an irregularly irregular rhythm. Abdominal examination reveals a soft, non-tender abdomen and normal bowel sounds. Neurological examination reveals expressive aphasia, left facial droop, right-sided sensory deficits, and right-sided motor strength of 3/5. Left arm and leg sensory and motor examination are normal.

Lab data show hemoglobin 12.6, hematocrit 38, WBCs 10,600, and platelets 186,000. Basic metabolic panel is normal. Point-of-care glucose is 109. CT scan of the head is normal.

1. What is the most likely diagnosis?
2. What is the most likely cause of this new diagnosis?
3. What else should be considered in the differential diagnosis?

Terminology in neurological department

disorder of consciousness 意识障碍
somnolence 嗜睡
sopor 昏睡状态

stupor 昏睡

coma 昏迷

confusion 意识模糊

twilight state 朦胧状态

delirium 谵妄

coma vigil 醒状昏迷

aphasia 失语症

apraxia 失用症

agnosis 失认症

vertigo 眩晕

dizziness 头晕

deafness 耳聋

tinnitus 耳鸣

hyperacusis 听觉过敏

syncope 晕厥

seizure 痫性发作

hyperesthesia 感觉过敏

dysestheisa 感觉迟钝

hyperpathia 感觉过度

paresthesia 感觉异常

paralysis 瘫痪

flaccid paralysis 弛缓性瘫痪

monoplegia 单瘫

spastic paralysis 痉挛性瘫痪

hemiplegia 偏瘫

paraplegia 截瘫

clasp-knife phenomenon 折刀样肌张力增高

pseudobulbar palsy 假性球麻痹、假性延髓麻痹

crossed hemiplegia 交叉性瘫痪

involuntary movement 不自主运动

static tremor 静止性震颤

lead-pipe rigidity 铅管样强直

cogwheel rigidity 齿轮样强直

chorea 舞蹈症

hemichorea 偏侧舞蹈症

athetosis 手足徐动症

dystonia 肌张力障碍

ataxia 共济失调

cerebellar ataxia 小脑共济失调

incoordination 协调运动障碍

vision disorder 视力障碍

sensory disorder 感觉障碍

nuchal rigidity (stiff neck) 颈强直

meningeal irritation 脑膜刺激征

Kernig sign 凯尔尼格征

Brudzinski sign 布鲁津斯基征

gag reflex 咽反射

oculocardiac reflex 眼心反射

carotid sinus reflex 颈动脉反射

pseudohypertrophy 假性肥大

muscular tension 肌张力

muscular power (force) 肌力

finger-to-nose test 指鼻试验

heel-to-knee test 跟膝胫试验

romberg sign 闭目难立征

gait 步态

spastic hemiplegic gait 痉挛性偏瘫步态

spastic paraparetic gait 痉挛性截瘫步态

festinating gait 慌张步态

drunken man gait 醉酒步态

gait of sensory ataxia 感觉性共济失调步态

steppage gait 跨阈步态

myopathic gait 肌病步态

hysterical gait 癔病步态

biceps reflex 肱二头肌反射

triceps reflex 肱三头肌反射

patellar tendon reflex 膝反射

achilles tendon reflex 踝反射

clonus 阵挛

Hoffmann sign 霍夫曼征

Rossolimo sign 罗索利莫征

abdominal reflexes 腹壁反射

cremasteric reflex 提睾反射

plantar reflex 跖反射

anal reflex 肛门反射

pathologic reflex 病理反射

Babinski sign 巴宾斯基征

Chaddock sign 查多克征

Oppenheim sign 奥本海姆征

Gordon sign 戈登征

Pussep sign 普塞征

opisthotonus 角弓反张

oculocephalic reflex 头眼反射

doll head test 玩偶头试验

vestibulo-ocular reflex 眼前庭反射

tonic neck reflex 紧张性颈反射

cerebrospinal fluid 脑脊液

diagnostic puncture 诊断性穿刺

lumbar puncture 腰椎穿刺

electroencephalography 脑电图

cerebral evoked potentials 脑诱发电位

electromyography 肌电图

biopsy of brain tissue 脑组织活检

trigeminal neuralgia 三叉神经痛

idiopathic facial palsy 特发性神经麻痹

hemifacial spasm 偏侧面肌痉挛

mononeuropathy 单神经病

carpal tunnel syndrome 腕管综合征

common peroneal nerve palsy 腓总神经麻痹

occipital neuralgia 枕神经痛

brachial neuralgia 臂神经痛

intercoastal neuralgia 肋间神经痛

lateral femoral cutaneous neuropathy 股外侧神经病

sciatica 坐骨神经痛

femoral neuralgia 股神经痛

polyneuropathy 多发性神经病

acute inflammatory demyelinating polyneuropathy 急性炎症性脱髓鞘性多发性神经病

Guillain-Barre syndrome 格林 - 巴利综合征

chronic inflammatory demyelinating polyneuropathy 慢性炎症性脱髓鞘性多发性神经病

acute myelitis 急性脊髓炎

acute transverse myelitis 急性横贯性脊髓炎

acute ascending myelitis 急性上升性脊髓炎

compressive myelopathy 脊髓压迫症

syringomyelia 脊髓空洞症

subacute combined degeneration of the spinal cord 脊髓亚急性联合变性

vascular diseases of the spinal cord 脊髓血管疾病

motor neuron diseases 运动神经元病

amyotrophic lateral sclerosis 肌萎缩性侧索硬化

progressive spinal muscular atrophy 进行性肌萎缩症

progressive bulbar palsy 进行性延髓麻痹

primary lateral sclerosis 原发性侧索硬化

spinal muscular atrophy 脊髓肌萎缩症

cerebrovascular disease 脑血管疾病

minor stroke 小卒中

major stroke 大卒中

silent stroke 静息性卒中

ischemic stroke 缺血性卒中

hemorrhagic stroke 出血性卒中

transient ischemic attack 短暂性脑缺血发作

cerebral infarction 脑梗死

cerebral ischemic stroke 缺血性脑卒中

cerebral thrombosis 脑血栓形成

reperfusion damage 再灌注损伤

cerebral watershed infarction 脑分水岭梗死

hemorrhagic infarction 出血性梗死

multiple infarction 多发性脑梗死

cerebral embolism 脑栓塞

intracerebral hemorrhage 脑出血

subarachnoid hemorrhage 蛛网膜下腔出血

hypertensive encephalopathy 高血压脑病

herpes simplex virus encephalitis 单纯性疱疹性脑炎

viral meningitis 病毒性脑膜炎

progressive multifocal leukoencephalopathy 进行性多灶性白质脑病

subacute sclerosing panencephalitis 亚急性硬化性全脑炎

tuberculous meningitis 结核性脑膜炎

neurosyphilis 神经梅毒

multiple sclerosis　多发性硬化

neuromyelitis optica　视神经脊髓炎

acute disseminated encephalomyelitis　急性播散性脑脊髓炎

movement disorder　运动障碍疾病

Parkinson's disease　帕金森病

essential tremor　特发性震颤

multiple tics-coprolalia syndrome　抽动秽语综合征

epilepsy　癫痫

migraine　偏头痛

tension headache　紧张性头痛

intracranial hypotension headache　低颅压性头痛

dementia　痴呆

Alzheimer disease　阿尔茨海默病

memory impairment　记忆障碍

cognitive impairment　认知障碍

vascular dementia　血管性痴呆

cerebral palsy　脑性瘫痪

congenital hydrocephalus　先天性脑积水

neurofibromatosis　神经纤维瘤病

tuberous sclerosis　结节性硬化症

myasthenia gravis　重症肌无力

progressive muscular dystrophy　进行性肌营养不良症

periodic paralysis　周期性瘫痪

polymyositis　多发性肌炎

myotonic dystrophy　强直性肌营养不良症

Chapter 7

Musculoskeletal System

Section A　Focus Listening

Conversation

Listen to the dialogue and fill in the blanks with proper words.

D=doctor P=patient

D: Hello, I'm Dr. Wang. Can you tell me what problem you have with your joints?

P: I got lots of pain in them.

D: Has the pain been getting worse recently?

P: Yes, over the past 3 months I have found the symptoms being deteriorated.

D: Which joints are mainly affected?

P: It involved my _____ interphalangeal joints.

D: Is there any time of day when your symptoms are worse?

P: Yes, I have joint stiffness in the morning when I get up.

D: How long did it last?

P: At least an hour, sometimes longer.

D: Have you noticed anything causing the symptoms worse?

P: Yes, the pain gets worse when I wash clothes or clean tableware in the cold water.

D: Do you remember whether there were any _____ symptoms before the proximal interphalangeal joints pain presented?

P: No, I was healthy until the finger joints pain presented.

D: Did it happen before this episode?

P: Yes, it's about 7-10 days ago, I could remember it clearly because my husband found me wasting.

D: Are there any other symptoms?

P: I had ____, malaise.

D: I need to examine your fingers now, please put your hand on the table.

P: OK.

D: Does it hurt when I press?

P: Yes, it hurts, and it also does when I flex my ____.

D: Yes, it's certain because your fingers are swollen.

P: Dr. Wang, what disease is it?

D: You're highly suspected to be suffered from rheumatoid arthritis. I'd like you to order some examination to evaluate the severity.

P: OK.

An hour later, the patient came back with results.

D: OK, let me have a look at these results… um, the routine blood test reveals:

Mild anemia, the erythrocyte sedimentation rate is 45 mm/h, which are twice higher than those of normal value and indicates higher activity and severity of synovitis, ____ factor: positive, serum complement 3 are significantly elevated. The plain radiograph shows: phalangeal soft tissue swelling, periarticular osteoporosis, marginal erosion, joint space narrowing. So you are diagnosed as rheumatoid arthritis. What tablets are you taking at present?

P: Only ibuprofen.

D: Ibuprofen is not enough at the moment, the treatment goals in rheumatoid arthritis are to control inflammatory diseases process and to prevent joint damage and normalize the functions of finger. Ibuprofen is used to kill pain. I'll prescribe methotrexate to control the disease process.

New Words & Expressions

interphalangeal 指节间的   phalangeal 指骨的

rheumatoid arthritis 类风湿性关节炎   anemia 贫血

erythrocyte 红细胞   sedimentation 沉降

synovitis 滑膜炎   radiograph X 光照片

methotrexate 甲氨蝶呤

Passage

Answer the questions after listening to the passage.

1. Which of the following substances is the toxin?

A. Tetanospasmin.   B. Tetanolysin.

C. Tetanus toxoid.   D. All of the above.

2. What is the name of the bacteria causing tetanus?

A. Clostridium perfringens.   B. Clostridium difficle.

C. Clostridium tetani.   D. Clostridium botulinum.

3. Which type of muscle is affected by tetanus?

A. Heart muscle.   B. Smooth muscle.

C. Skeletal muscle.   D. All of the above.

4. Which language is the term tetanus derived from?

A. Arabic.   B. Latin.   C. Chinese.   D. Greek.

5. Which of the following is NOT true regarding tetanus?

A. It is caused by bacteria.

B. Skeletal muscles are affected.

C. Heart muscles are affected.

D.Tetanus toxin inhibits the release of inhibitory neurotransmitter.

Section B   Reading Comprehension

Text

I was asked to see a 76-year-old Japanese-American woman with Takayasu arteritis, a diagnosis first examined in 1984, when at age 33 years, she was found to have multiple arterial bruits. At the time, the patient had a normal erythrocyte sedimentation rate (ESR), and her arteritis appeared to be inactive and did not require steroids. In fact, she has never been treated with steroids for Takayasu arteritis.

In 1989, MRI examination of the chest showed a proximal ascending aorta rotation with a constant diameter of 4 cm, which has remained at that size until now. The descending aorta was normal, and there was no evidence of dissection or aneurysm.

The patient had been seen by many specialists in Japan, some of whom believed she had Takayasu arteritis and others who believed her vascular abnormalities were caused by atherosclerosis, perhaps related to her MTHFR gene status. The patient was also found to have mild aortic insufficiency; but, aside from when she suffered a saddle pulmonary embolism in 2016, the patient denied chest pain or shortness of breath, and there was no claudication-type symptoms in the arms and legs. She didn't have cerebrovascular accidents but did have a hemorrhage in the right eye.

ESR during the pulmonary embolism episode in September 2016 was 55 mm/hour; in March 2017, the ESR was 70 mm/hour; and today it is normal at 17 mm/hour with a normal

C-reactive protein. The patient had a history of trigger fingers, knee osteoarthritis, low back pain, and osteoporosis. At no time, she had joint inflammation, stiffness or fatigue, and she denied a history of Raynaud phenomenon, skin rash, hemoptysis, fever, or weight loss.

Physical Examination

The patient's vital signs were normal with equal blood pressures in arms and legs. Loud bilateral carotid and subclavian bruits were heard and radial pulses were barely palpable. No ischemic arm or leg findings were noted.

Laboratory Tests—May 10, 2016

- Comprehensive chemistry panel: glucose, 148 mg/dL, creatinine, 0.9 mg/dL
- Normal complete blood count
- Urinalysis, 1+ blood but only 1 red blood cell
- Spot urine protein/creatinine ratio, 6/33.7, 180 mg/g
- Cyclic citrullinated peptide antibodies negative
- Rheumatoid factor negative
- Anti-Ro, 77 U (normal <20), anti-La, anti-Sm, anti-RNP, all negative
- Antithyroglobulin, 114 IU/mL (normal <4.11), antithyroid peroxidase, 113 IU/mL (normal <5.61)
- Antinuclear antibody negative, anti-double-stranded DNA negative

MRI

The patient underwent aortic MRI angiography on March 10, 2016, and a chest MRI without and with contrast on March 28, 2017.

She had a left-sided aortic arch with a normal branching pattern of the great vessels. There was no evidence of thoracic aortic dissection or coarctation. Irregular mural thickening was noted at the level of the aortic arch, great vessels, and throughout the descending thoracic aorta, but overall, no significant changes were noted. There were stable stenosis at the origin and proximal right brachiocephalic artery and proximal right common carotid artery. The thoracic aorta appeared normal in size.

Views of the left ventricle were very limited; however, normal size and systolic function were demonstrated. Her aortic valve was trileaflet, and she has mild aortic regurgitation and no significant aortic stenosis.

Impressions:

1. No significant interval change was seen in the appearance of the irregular mural thickening of the aortic arch, great vessels, and throughout the descending thoracic aorta.

2. Stable stenosis of the right brachiocephalic artery and proximal right common carotid artery were noted.

3. No evidence was seen of thoracic aortic aneurysm, dissection, or coarctation.

4. The aortic valve is trileaflet with mild aortic regurgitation.

New Words & Expressions

takayasu *n.* 大动脉炎

arteritis [ˈɑ:təraɪtɪs] *n.* inflammation of an artery 动脉炎

erythrocyte [ɪˈrɪθrəsaɪt] *n.* also called red blood cell 红细胞

sedimentation [ˌsedɪmenˈteɪʃn] *n.* the natural process by which small pieces of rock, earth etc settle at the bottom of the water or sea and form a solid layer 沉降；沉积

proximal [ˈprɒksɪməl] *a.* situated close to the centre, median line, or point of attachment or origin 近中心的

aorta [eɪˈɔ:tə] *n.* the large trunk artery that carries blood from the left ventricle of the heart to branch arteries 主动脉

pulmonary [ˈpʌlmənəri] *a.* relating to or affecting the lungs 肺的；有肺的；肺状的

embolism [ˈembəlɪzəm] *n.* something such as a hard mass of blood or a small amount of air that blocks a tube carrying blood through the body 栓塞；血栓

claudication [ˌklɔdəˈkeɪʃən] *n.* disability of walking due to crippling of the legs or feet 跛行；跛

cerebrovascular [ˌserəbrəʊˈvæskjələ] *a.* of or relating to the blood vessels and the blood supply of the brain 脑血管的

hemorrhage [ˈhemərɪdʒ] *n.* flow of blood from a ruptured blood vessels 出血（等于 haemorrhage）

osteoarthritis [ˌɒstiəʊɑ:ˈθraɪtɪs] *n.* chronic breakdown of cartilage in the joints; the most common form of arthritis occurring usually after middle age 骨关节炎

hemoptysis [hɪˈmɑptəsɪs] *n.* coughing up blood from the respiratory tract; usually indicates a severe infection of the bronchioles lungs 咳血

bilateral [ˌbaɪˈlætərəl] *a.* having two sides or parts 两边的

subclavian [sʌbˈkleviən] *a.* (of an artery, vein, area, etc) situated below the clavicle （动脉，血管，区域等）锁骨下的

palpable [ˈpælpəbl] *a.* capable of being perceived by the senses or the mind; especially capable of being handled or touched or felt 可触知的；易觉察的

ischemic [ɪsˈkimɪk] *a.* 缺血性的；局部缺血的

citrullinated *n.* 瓜氨酸化

rheumatoid [ˈrʊmətɔɪd] *a.* (of the symptoms of a disease) resembling rheumatism 类风湿的

antithyroglobulin [əntɪθaɪrəʊgˈləʊbjʊlɪn] *n.* 抗甲状腺球蛋白

thoracic [θəˈræsɪk] *a.* of or relating to the chest or thorax 胸的；胸廓的

stenosis [stɪˈnəʊsɪs] *n.* an abnormal narrowing of a bodily canal or passage （器官）狭窄症

---

brachiocephalic [breɪkɪəsɪˈfælɪk] *a.* of, relating to, or supplying the arm and head 头臂的；支持头臂的

regurgitation [riˌɡəːdʒiˈteiʃən] *n.* backflow of blood through a defective heart valve 回流

Exercise

Decide whether the following statements are true (T) or false (F) according to the passage.

_____1. When the doctor was asked to see the patient, she had a normal erythrocyte sedimentation rate, and her arteritis seemed not to be active and did not need steroids.

_____2. The patient denied any cerebrovascular accident but did have a hemorrhage in the left eye.

_____3. The patient has had a history of trigger fingers, knee osteoarthritis, right back pain, and osteoporosis.

_____4. The patient had a left-sided aortic arch with a normal branching pattern of the great vessels in her recent MRI.

_____5. In the patient's impressions, stable stenosis of the right brachiocephalic artery and proximal left common carotid artery were noted.

Answer the following questions according to the passage.

1. What probably made the specialists have different diagnosis when the patient had been seen by many specialists in Japan?

_____

2. What appeared in the patient's physical examination?

_____

3. Based on the impressions, what probable treatment do you make?

_____

Use the appropriate form of the words or phrases in the box to complete the following sentences.

erythrocyte	rheumatoid	common	ischemic	bilateral
ascend	claudication	takayasu	fatigue	aneurysm
pulmonary	citrullinated	hemorrhage		

1. He reportedly had dried blood around his mouth and nose and bruising on his chest, suggesting a massive _____ brought on by tuberculosis.

2. They suspect he is suffering from a _____ embolism, basically a blood clot in an artery of the lung that could prove fatal.

3. These results explained that increasing on aggregation and coagulation of blood, decreasing on _____'s deformability.

4. An abdominal aortic _____ is a weakened and bulging area in the lower part of the aorta, the major blood vessel that supplies blood to the body.

5. Drinking alcohol may reduce the pain, stiffness, and joint damage caused by _____ _____ arthritis, reports a new research.

6. Initially patients may be able to walk through the pain, but as the disease progresses further, this is not possible and the _____ pain causes limping and can only relieved by resting.

7. We need to build trust with the Russians on _____ security matters — relations, one on one.

8. A slow and steady trek that allows times for acclimatization is the safest way to _____ and prevent altitude sickness, which could have fatal consequences.

9. Let us find that _____ stake we all have in one another, and let our politics reflect that spirit as well.

10. If you feel acute soreness or have lingering _____, progress to the next week's training only when you can comfortably complete the preceding week's goal.

Translation

A. Translate the following expressions into English.

1. 轻度主动脉瓣返流　　　　　2. 胸主动脉夹层动脉瘤
3. 收缩功能　　　　　　　　　4. 重度主动脉瓣闭锁不全
5. 红细胞沉降率　　　　　　　6. 环瓜氨酸多肽抗体
7. 跛行类症状　　　　　　　　8. 基因状态

B. Translate the following sentences into Chinese.

1. The descending aorta was normal, and there was no evidence of dissection or aneurysm.

2. No significant interval change was seen in the appearance of the irregular mural thickening of the aortic arch, great vessels, and throughout the descending thoracic aorta.

3. At no time she had joint inflammation, stiffness, or fatigue, and she denies a history of Raynaud phenomenon, skin rash, hemoptysis, fever, or weight loss.

4. Irregular mural thickening was noted at the level of the aortic arch, great vessels, and throughout the descending thoracic aorta, but overall, no significant changes were noted.

5. Loud bilateral carotid and subclavian bruits were heard and radial pulse was barely palpable.

Section C   Vocabulary (Terminology)

1. 钙 calcium

Combining form	Meaning	Terminology	Terminology meaning
calc/o	calcium	hypercalcemia	an excess of calcium in the blood 高血钙症
calci/o	calcium	decalcification	the removal or loss of calcium or calcium compounds (as from bones or soil) 脱钙

2. 骨 bone, os(拉丁语)

Combining form	Meaning	Terminology	Terminology meaning
oste/o	bone	osteoarthritis	arthritis marked by degeneration of the cartilage and bone of joints 骨关节炎

3. 软骨 cartilage

Combining form	Meaning	Terminology	Terminology meaning
chondro	cartilage	chondrosarcoma	软骨瘤

4. 颅骨 cranium

Combining form	Meaning	Terminology	Terminology meaning
crani/o	cranium (skull bones)	craniotomy	surgical opening of the skull 颅骨切开术

5. 上颌骨 maxilla, upper jaw bone

Combining form	Meaning	Terminology	Terminology meaning
maxilla/o	maxilla	maxillary	of or relating to maxilla 上颌骨的

6. 下颌骨 mandible, lower jaw bone

Combining form	Meaning	Terminology	Terminology meaning
mandibu/o	mandible	mandibular	of or relating to mandible 下颌骨的

7. 脊椎骨 vertebra

Combining form	Meaning	Terminology	Terminology meaning
spondyl/o	vertebra	spondylosis	椎关节强硬
vertebr/o		vertebral	of, relating to, or being vertebrae or the vertebral column 椎骨的，脊椎的

8. 锁骨 clavicle, collar bone

Combining form	Meaning	Terminology	Terminology meaning
clavicul/o	clavicle, collar bone	supraclavicular	above the clavicle 锁骨上的 supra-means above

9. 胸骨 sternum

Combining form	Meaning	Terminology	Terminology meaning
stern/o	sternum	sternocleido mastoid	胸锁乳突的

10. 肋骨 ribs

Combining form	Meaning	Terminology	Terminology meaning
cost/o	ribs	subcostal	below the ribs 肋骨下的

11. 髂骨 ilium（upper part pelvic bone）

Combining form	Meaning	Terminology	Terminology meaning
ili/o	ilium (upper part pelvic bone)	iliac	of, relating to, or located near the ilium 髂骨的

12. 坐骨 ischium, posterior part of pelvic bone

Combining form	Meaning	Terminology	Terminology meaning
isch/o	ischium	ischial	of, relating to ischium 坐骨的

13. 股骨 femur, thigh bone

Combining form	Meaning	Terminology	Terminology meaning
femor/o	femur, thigh bone	femoral	of or relating to the femur or thigh 股骨的

14. 膝盖骨 patella, kneecap

Combining form	Meaning	Terminology	Terminology meaning
patell/o	patella, kneecap	subpatellar	below the patella 膝盖骨下的

15. 胫骨 tibia, shin bone

Combining form	Meaning	Terminology	Terminology meaning
tibi/o	tibia, shin bone	tibial	of or relating to tibia 胫骨的

16. 腓骨 fibula

Combining form	Meaning	Terminology	Terminology meaning
perone/o	fibula	peroneal	of, relating to, or located near the fibula 腓骨的
fibul/o	fibula (small lower leg bone)	fibular	of, relating to, or located near the fibula 腓骨的

17. 跟骨 heel bone, calcaneus

Combining form	Meaning	Terminology	Terminology meaning
calcane/o	heel bone, calcaneus	calcaneal	relating to the heel or calcaneus 跟骨的

18. 跗骨 tarsals

Combining form	Meaning	Terminology	Terminology meaning
tars/o	tarsals(bones of the hindfoot)	tarsectomy	跗骨切除术

19. 跖骨 metatarsals, foot bone

Combining form	Meaning	Terminology	Terminology meaning
metatars/o	metatarsals	metatarsalgia	跖骨痛

20. 指趾骨 phalanx (pl:phalanges,finger and/or toe bones)

Combining form	Meaning	Terminology	Terminology meaning
phalang/o	phalanges	phalangeal	of or relating to a phalanx or the phalanges 指趾的

21. 肩胛骨 scapula, shoulder bone

Combining form	Meaning	Terminology	Terminology meaning
scapula/o	scapula, shoulder bone	scapular	of or relating to the shoulder, the scapula, or scapulars 肩胛（骨）的；肩的

22. 肱骨 humerus

Combining form	Meaning	Terminology	Terminology meaning
humer/o	humerus	humeral	of, relating to, or situated in the region of the humerus or shoulder 肱骨的

23. 尺骨 ulna

Combining form	Meaning	Terminology	Terminology meaning
uln/o	ulna (lower arm bone- little finger side)	ulnar	of, relating to the ulna 尺骨的

24. 桡骨 radius

Combining form	Meaning	Terminology	Terminology meaning
radi/o	radius(lower arm-thumb side)	radial	of, relating to the radius 桡骨的

25. 腕 carpal, wrist bone

Combining form	Meaning	Terminology	Terminology meaning
carp/o	carpal, wrist bone	carpal	of, relating to the carpal 腕骨的

26. 掌骨 metacarpal, hand bone

Combining form	Meaning	Terminology	Terminology meaning
metacarp/o	metacarpal	metacarpectomy	removal of metacarpals 掌骨切除术

27. 关节 joint

Combining form	Meaning	Terminology	Terminology meaning
arthr/o	joint	arthropathy	a disease of a joint 关节病
articul/o		articular cartilage	关节软骨

28. 韧带 ligament

Combining form	Meaning	Terminology	Terminology meaning
ligament/o	ligament	ligamentous	of or relating the ligament 韧带的

29. 肌腱 tendon

Combining form	Meaning	Terminology	Terminology meaning
ten/o	tendon	tenorrhaphy	肌腱缝合
tendin/o	tendon	tendonitis	inflammation of a tendon 肌腱炎

30. 滑膜 synovial membrane

Combining form	Meaning	Terminology	Terminology meaning
synov/o	synovial membrane	synovitis	inflammation of a synovial membrane 滑膜炎

31. 囊，黏液囊

Combining form	Meaning	Terminology	Terminology meaning
burs/o	bursa	bursitis	inflammation of a bursa (as of the shoulder or elbow) 黏液囊炎

32. 肌肉 muscle

Combining form	Meaning	Terminology	Terminology meaning
my/o	muscle	eletromyography	an instrument that converts the electrical activity associated with functioning skeletal muscle into a visual record or into sound and is used to diagnose neuromuscular disorders and in biofeedback training 肌电图描记器
myos/o		myositis	soreness of voluntary muscle due to inflammation 肌炎

33. 僵直，僵硬 stiff

Combining form	Meaning	Terminology	Terminology meaning
ankyl/o	stiff	ankylosis	stiffness or fixation of a joint by disease or surgery 关节僵硬

34. 不成熟细胞 embryonic or immature cell

Combining form	Meaning	Terminology	Terminology meaning
-blast	embryonic or immature cell	osteoblast	a bone-forming cell 成骨细胞

35. 破裂，破碎 break

Combining form	Meaning	Terminology	Terminology meaning
-clast	to break	osteoclast	any of the large multinucleate cells closely associated with areas of bone resorption 破骨细胞

36. 滑动，滑行 slipping

Combining form	Meaning	Terminology	Terminology meaning
-listhesis	slipping	spondylolisthesis	脊椎前移

37. 软化 softening

Combining form	Meaning	Terminology	Terminology meaning
-malacia	softening	osteomalacia	a disease of adults that is characterized by softening of the bones and is analogous to rickets in the young 软骨病

38. 生长 grow

Combining form	Meaning	Terminology	Terminology meaning
-physis	to grow	epiphysis	a part or process of a bone that ossified separately and later becomes ankylosed to the main part of the bone; especially : an end of a long bone 骺

39. 空洞形成 pore, passage

Combining form	Meaning	Terminology	Terminology meaning
-porosis	pore, passage	osteoporosis	a condition that affects especially older women and is characterized by decrease in bone mass with decreased density and enlargement of bone spaces producing porosity and fragility 骨质疏松症

40. 刀，片，层 instrument to cut

Combining form	Meaning	Terminology	Terminology meaning
-tome	instrument to cut	osteotome	骨刀（凿）

41. 固定，固定术 to bind, tie together

Combining form	Meaning	Terminology	Terminology meaning
-desis	to bind, tie together	arthrodesis	the surgical immobilization of a joint so that the bones grow solidly together 关节固定术

42. 狭窄 narrowing

Combining form	Meaning	Terminology	Terminology meaning
-stenosis	narrowing	spinal stenosis	椎管狭窄

43. 筋膜 fascia

Combining form	Meaning	Terminology	Terminology meaning
fasci/o	fascia(forms sheaths enveloping muscle)	fasciectomy	筋膜切除术

44. 纤维组织 fibrous connective tissue

Combining form	Meaning	Terminology	Terminology meaning
fibr/o	fibrous connective tissue	fibromyalgia	any of a group of rheumatic disorders affecting soft tissues and characterized by pain, tenderness, and stiffness of muscles and associated connective tissue structures 纤维肌痛

45. 平滑肌 smooth muscle

Combining form	Meaning	Terminology	Terminology meaning
leiomy/o	smooth muscle	leiomyoma	平滑肌瘤

46. 足底 sole of the foot

Combining form	Meaning	Terminology	Terminology meaning
plant/o	sole of the foot	plantar flexion	of or relating to the sole of the foot 足底的

47. 横纹肌 skeletal muscle

Combining form	Meaning	Terminology	Terminology meaning
rhabdomy/o	skeletal muscle	rhabdomyosarcoma	a malignant tumor composed of striated muscle fibers 横纹肌肉瘤

48. 虚弱 lack of strength, weakness

Combining form	Meaning	Terminology	Terminology meaning
-asthenia	lack of strength, weakness	myasthenia	muscular debility 肌无力

49. 发育，营养 development, nourishment

Combining form	Meaning	Terminology	Terminology meaning
-trophy	development, nourishment	atrophy	decrease in size or wasting away of a body part or tissue 萎缩

50. 偏离，离开 away from

Combining form	Meaning	Terminology	Terminology meaning
ab-	away from	abduction	the action of abducting 外展

51. 运动，方向，变化，增加，靠近 toward

Combining form	Meaning	Terminology	Terminology meaning
ad-	toward	adduction	the action of adducting 内收

52. 背 back

Combining form	Meaning	Terminology	Terminology meaning
dorsi-	back	dorsiflexion	背屈

53. 多 many, much

Combining form	Meaning	Terminology	Terminology meaning
poly-	many,much	polymyalgia rheumatica	it is a syndrome marked by aching and morning stiffness in the shoulder hip, or neck for more than one month 风湿性多肌痛

Exercise for vocabulary

Match the following pathological condition or terms with their meaning below.

osteomalacia	tendonitis	abduction	arthrodesis	iliac
femoral	myasthenia	osteoarthritis	humeral	radial
osteoporosis	synovitis	osteoclast	ankyloses	myalgia
osteoblast	hypertrophy	arthropathy	adduction	rheumatoid
arthritis				

_____1. Inflammation of a synovial membrane

_____2. Of or relating to the femur or thigh

_____3. Muscular debility

_____4. Excessive development of an organ or part

_____5. The action of abducting

_____6. A disease of a joint

_____7. Pain in one or more muscles

_____8. A bone-forming cell

_____9. Inflammation of a tendon

_____10. A disease of adults that is characterized by softening of the bones and is analogous to rickets in the young

_____11. Inflammation of bone

_____12. Arthritis marked by degeneration of the cartilage and bone of joints

_____13. The action of adducting

_____14. The surgical immobilization of a joint so that the bones grow solidly together

_____15. Any of the large multinucleate cells closely associated with areas of bone resorption

_____16. Of, relating to, or situated in the region of the humerus or shoulder

_____17. Of, relating to the radius

_____18. Stiffness or fixation of a joint by disease or surgery

_____19. A condition that affects especially older women and is characterized by decrease in bone mass with decreased density and enlargement of bone spaces producing porosity and fragility

_____20. Of, relating to, or located near the ilium

Choose the term that best completes the meaning of the sentence.

1. Mr. Xie, male, aged 48, had been complaining of wrist pain with tingling sensations in his fingers for months. Chief Dr. Zhong diagnosed his condition as _____.

A. osteomyelitis   B. rheumatoid arthritis

C. carpal tunnel syndrome   D. nerve injury

2. Ms. Liu, aged 59, was admitted to orthopedic department on Feb. 6th, 2016 because of femoral neck fracture for half an hour, she stated she had back pain for over 2 years, she had noticed loss of height and kyphosis. And the radiographs reveal: osteopenia, loss of horizontal vertebral trabeculation. Dr. Liang diagnosed her condition as _____ except femoral neck fracture.

A. osteoporosis   B. osteoarthritis

C. hypertrophic osteoarthropathy   D. rheumatoid arthritis

3. Miss Xiong, aged 19, complains morning stiffness in symmetric fingers for over 2 months. There were pain and swelling in fingers on exercises, it didn't alleviated after being treated with aspirin and other NASDs, however the condition is getting worse, and fatigue, poor appetite, loss of weight, irregular fever presented, blood test shows rheumatoid factor: 2+, so the probable diagnosis is _____?

A. rheumatoid arthritis   B. rheumatic arthritis

C. gout   D. peptic ulcer

4. Ms. Xiao, aged 19, complains remittent fever for 7 days, 2 days ago she found the symmetric and swollen erythema presented, she stated pain in several joints, fever and malaise, laboratory findings show: HB 90g/L, WBC 3.4×10^9/L, urinalysis shows: proteinuria, ANA: positive, SLE: positive. What is the mostly like diagnosis?

A. Polyarthritis.   B. Lyme disease.

C. Ankylosing spondylitis.   D. Leukemia.

5. Ms Li, female, aged 10, complained of pyrexia with sore throat and pain in knee, wrist and ankle joints for 1 week, on examination: congestive pharynx, II degree tonsillar swelling, the cardiac and pulmonary examinations are within normal limits, swelling and redness and significant tenderness in knee joints. The laboratory findings show: WBC

$18.2 \times 10^9/L$, anti-streptolysin "O":1:1250/mL, ANA: positive, what's the mostly like diagnosis?

A. Systemic lupus erythematosus.   B. Rheumatoid arthritis.

C. Rheumatic arthritis.   D. Leukocytosis.

6. A 40-year-old female states pain and swelling in both wrists and knees for seven weeks. The patient complains of fatigue and lethargy several weeks before noticing the joint pain. The patient notes that after a period of rest, resistance to movement is more striking, on exam the metacarpophalangeal joints and wrists are warm and tender. There are no other joint abnormalities. There is no alopecia, photosensitivity, kidney disease, or rash. Which of the following is correct?

A. The clinical picture suggests early rheumatoid arthritis, and a rheumatoid factor should be obtained.

B. Lack of systemic suggests osteoarthritis.

C. The prodrome of lethargy suggests chronic fatigue syndrome.

D. She can be diagnosed as degenerative osteoarthropathy.

7. Selma, a 40-year-old secretary, had been complaining of wrist pain with tingling sensation in her fingers for months. Dr. Ayres diagnosed her condition as_____.

A. osteomyelitis   B. rheumatoid arthritis

C. carpal tunnel syndrome   D. muscle injury

8. Daisy tripped while playing tennis and landed on her hand. She had excruciating pain and a _____fracture that required casting.

A. Ewing   B. colles

C. pathological   D. shoulder-hand syndrome

9. In her fifties, Estelle started hunching over more and more. Her doctor realized that she was developing _____and prescribed to repair ligaments.

A. gout arthritis   B. osteoarthritis   C. osteoporosis   D. aging

10. Paul had a skiing accident and ligaments were tore in his knee. Dr. Miller recommended _____ to repair the ligaments.

A. electromyography   B. hypertrophy

C. arthroscopic surgery   D. pain killers

Section D Writing

Medications（药物史）

药物史 (Medications, Meds) 包括所有现在和近期的药物使用情况，还包括任何药店购买的非处方药和偶尔使用的中草药制剂。另外，要求列出所有药物剂量、给药途径及用药间隔时间，包括非处方药以及近期停用、改变用法的药物。如果近期改变剂量，也应说明。多数情况下，使用药物商品名或化学名均可。

Example:

1. Lisinopril 10 mg po qd
2. Lanoxin 0.125mg po qd
3. Vitamin B$_{12}$ 100μg im q month
4. Pravastatin 40 mg (increased from 20 mg 3 weeks ago) poqn
5. Multivitamin 1 po qd
6. St. John's wort (dose unkown) 1 tablet po qd prn depressed mood

1. 赖诺普利 10mg，口服，每日 1 次
2. 地高辛 0.125mg，口服，每日 1 次
3. 维生素 B$_{12}$ 100μg，肌肉注射，每月 1 次
4. 普伐他汀 400mg（3 周前从 20mg 增加至目前剂量），口服，每晚 1 次
5. 复合维生素，一片，口服，每日 1 次
6. 金丝桃（剂量不详），情绪低落的状态下必要时口服，1 片，每日 1 次

Exercise: Write the following medications.

1. 叔丁喘宁，吸入，每日 3 次
2. 氨茶碱片 1 片，口服，每日 3 次
3. 咳必清 25mg，口服，每日 3 次
4. 必嗽平 16mg，口服，每日 3 次
5. 头孢拉定 0.5g，口服，每日 3 次
6. 维生素 C 0.2g，口服，每日 3 次

Allergies（过敏史）

过敏史是病历中最重要的部分之一。医生需要亲自确认过敏反应并询问患者对所药物有什么反应。另外，询问患者是否在服用其他同类药物对鉴别药物过敏反应和不良反应非常重要。例如：有些患者声称对青霉素过敏，却可以服用阿莫西林。所以应将这些药物归类为"不能耐受药物"，而不能将其记录为过敏药物。需要特别提醒的是，过敏史不包括季节性过敏、花粉症、接触性过敏反应，这些都属于既往史范畴。

过敏史（allergies）则要求列出患者所有曾有反应的药物并列出药物反应。

Example:

1. Sulfa drug — rash
2. Ampicillin — anaphylaxis

例：

1. 磺胺药—皮疹
2. 氨苄西林—过敏反应

Exercise: Write the following allergy

请按过敏史书写格式完成某患者的过敏史：
1. 红霉素—皮疹、药物热、嗜酸粒细胞增多
2. 头孢曲松钠—恶心，呼吸困难，皮炎

Family History

家族史（family history, FHx）记录患者近亲和配偶的健康情况，要求列出或以图表表示家族成员及每一个家族成员的主要疾病和已故成员的死因。

家族成员主要是指父母、亲兄弟姊妹、子女和配偶。有时也涉及祖父母、外祖父母及其兄弟姊妹。

家族成员的健康情况一般介绍是否健在，是否有或有过遗传病、传染病（主要是指肝炎、发病、艾滋病），如有死亡，说明死因及时间。

家族史的重要性在于有助于明确某些疾病的危险因素——家族性或暴露相关的危险因素。本部分可以用词组、短句，甚至可以用上述的家族图谱表示，并把适当的疾病诊断名称写在代表家族成员的圆圈或方框下面。我们先学习一些常用词语，再看家族史书写例子。

常用词语：
一般健康情况：
in bad/poor health, unhealthy 不健康
healthy, in good health 健康
be living and well 健在
be alive 活着
die, be dead 死亡

常见句型：
1. … be living and well./ … be in good health./ … be well with no evidence of... illness.
His parents, wife and two children are living and well.
他的父母均健在，妻子和两个孩子健康。

2. There is no family history of (disease). /there was no (disease) in one's family.
His wife and two children are in good health, there is no family history of tuberculosis.
他的妻子和两个孩子健康，无结核病家族史。

3. There was no case of (disease) in one's family. No one in her/his family experienced (disease).
There was no case of cancer in her family.

她的家族成员没患过癌症。

4. Family history showed/revealed …

Family history showed tuberculosis in his both parents.

他的父母均患过结核病。

5. There was a family /hereditary tendency to … /there was a strong family history of … / there was a high incidence of … in the family.

There was a high incidence of hemophilia in his family. Four members of his generation were affected.

家族中血友病发病率很高。他这一代就有 4 人患过此病。

6. There was a high prevalence of … in the family.

There was a high prevalence of pulmonary cancer in his family.

他家族中肺癌的患病率较高。

7. … was irrelevant to …

His family history was irrelevant to his present illness.

他的家族成员中无人与他的现有疾病有关。

8. positive for some disease in someone.

Positive for cardiac failure in his grandfather.

他祖父患过心力衰竭。

9. … as a family characteristic.

The patient recognized that obesity was a peculiar characteristic of his family.

他认为肥胖是他家族的一个特点。

10. … die of … (a disease, old age, poison)/ … died from (a wound, overwork, etc.) … / died at the age of …

The patient's father died of apoplexy at the age of 76.

患者的父亲死于中风，享年 76 岁。

11. … (someone's) death was due to …

His brother's death was due to a car accident.

他的兄弟死于车祸。

Example:

Family history: The patient is youngest of 3 children. He has 2 older brothers, one 34 and the other 36. The 36-year-old one was diagnosed last year with hypertension, and the 34-year-old one has lupus and vitiligo. The patient's mother died of lung cancer in 1997. The patient's father has had skin cancer removed (type unknown) and is being treated for depression and anxiety. No information is available about grandparents. The patient denies a family history of diabetes, non-melanoma skin cancers, thyroid diseases, myocardial infarctions, or strokes.

家族史：患者是 3 个孩子中最小的一个。他有两个哥哥，一个 34 岁，一个 36

岁，36 岁的长兄去年确诊患有高血压，另一位 34 岁的兄长患有狼疮和白癜风。患者母亲于 1997 死于肺癌。患者父亲患有皮肤癌，已手术切除（病理类型不详），并患有抑郁症和焦虑症，现治疗中。患者祖父母的健康情况不详。患者否认家族性糖尿病史、非黑色素瘤皮肤癌病史、甲状腺疾病史、心肌梗死史和卒中史。

Exercise: Write the following family history.

1. 家族史：患者父亲死于肺癌，性质不详。母亲死于冠状动脉血栓形成。患者的妻子及三个孩子均体健。家族中无结核病史。母亲家族糖尿病史明显。

2. 家族史：患者父母及一兄健在，家族中无类似患者，无遗传性及家族性疾病患者。

Social History, SHx

社会活动史一般包括：
1. 职业、嗜好、个人兴趣
2. 婚姻状况、子女数目、社会支持网络和生活状况
3. 烟酒嗜好和违禁药物使用情况
4. 性生活史

与家族史一样，不同医生对社会活动史的写法有明显的不同。典型的社会活动史包括患者职业（包括重要的暴露史，例如化学药物、粉尘和放射线暴露史）、个人嗜好、婚姻状况、生育史、家庭成员、社会支持网络和生活状态，以及患者出生地和既往生活的地方。个人嗜好，比如吸烟、饮酒、药物使用和性生活等也需要包括在内。有的医生认为应将这部分内容划分为社会活动史、职业史、个人嗜好，如何取舍完全取决于医生个人。

Example 1

Social history: The patient was employed as a meat packer during his 30s and 40s and recently left that to join his brother doing construction. He does lay insulation but has not known asbestos exposure and wears an industrial mask. His only chemical exposure is to paint thinner. He got married at 22 years old and lives with his wife and three children in Chelsea in a single family home. He enjoys coaching little league baseball and is taking a correspondence course to get his bachelor's degree. He denies cigarette use but admits to consume 2–3 units of alcohol once or twice weekly with friends (CAGE questions 0 of 4). He denies illicit drug use and has had a monogamous sexual relationship with his wife since they got married.

例 1

社会史：患者在 30 ～ 40 岁时从事肉食品包装工作，近来转行与自己兄弟一起从事建筑业。患者从事放置绝缘材料的工作，但没有明确的石棉暴露史，作业时戴工业口罩，唯一的化学暴露为油漆稀释剂。患者 22 岁结婚，与妻子及 3 个孩子居

住在切尔西。患者曾兼任小联盟棒球队教练工作，并正在进行学士学位的函授课程学习。患者不吸烟，平时每周和朋友聚会 1～2 次，一起饮酒 2～3 个酒精单位，无不良嗜好，无非法药物滥用史。患者自结婚以来，仅与他妻子发生性关系。

Example 2

SHx: Married at 27 years old with 1 child

　　　Taking course to get to Ph.D

　　　Chief of No.2 hosptial

OccHx: Does medical work

　　　 No dangerous exposure

Habits: Denies tobacco and illicit drug use

　　　Admits to 2~3 bottle beer every day

　　　CAGE questions 0 of 4

　　　Monogamous relationship with wife since married.

例 2

社会活动史：27 岁结婚，育有 1 子

　　　　　　攻读博士学位

　　　　　　第二医院院长

职业史：从事医疗工作

　　　　无危险品接触史

个人嗜好：否认吸烟和非法药物使用

　　　　　每日 3 瓶啤酒

　　　　　无不良嗜好

　　　　　自结婚以来，妻子是其唯一的性伴侣

第二个病例使用了更多的短句结构，这是社会活动史的另一种书写风格。

Section E　Spoken English

Role play

Directions: A patient felt pain in the shoulder and could not wash face for two months. The patient went to clinic for help. Two students work in pairs to demonstrate the conversation, one plays the role of doctor, the other of patient.

Discussion

Directions: Work in groups and discuss with your partners, then answer the following questions with detailed analysis.

An 80-year-old female is admitted to the hospital following a fall on an icy side-walk. She suffered a left intertrochanteric hip fracture. There was no loss of consciousness or other injury. She was promptly transported to the ED for evaluation. Her primary physician admitted her, completed a preoperative risk assessment, and consulted the orthopedic surgery service after finding her to be suitable to undergo the risk of an orthopedic procedure. She has a history of well-controlled hypertension. She has no history of diabetes mellitus, coronary artery disease, kidney disease, congestive heart failure, or stroke. She is a nonsmoker, does not consume alcohol, and has no allergies. She takes hydrochlorothiazide 25 mg daily and atenolol 50mg daily. She had an appendectomy 40 years ago without complication. She is widowed, lives independently, and completes her activities of daily living, including light housework and climbing even one stair. She drives and manages her own finances.

The orthopedic surgery service surgically repaired the fracture with an open reduction and internal fixation. She was generally well tolerated with spinal anesthesia. She is now on the medical-surgical floor. The orthopedic surgery resident called and asked you manage her pain and hypertension. She is otherwise following routine postoperative orthopedic protocol for venous thromboembolism (VTE) prophylaxis, activity, diet, and wound care. The patient states her pain severity was 8 out of 10 during your evaluation.

Physical examination reveals a 5-ft 2-in, 52-kg (BMI 21) elderly caucasian female in moderate distress from pain. Her pulse is 100 bpm and regular, BP is 150/90 mm Hg, RR is 20/min, and temperature is 37℃ . Her skin is warm and dry and with good capillary refill. Chest is clear to auscultation bilaterally with good inspiratory effort. Cardiac examination reveals tachycardia with a regular rhythm. S1 and S2 are noted without murmurs. Abdomen has normal bowel sounds and is non-tender to palpation. Extremities show good pulses in all extremities with no edema. The left hip surgical dressing is intact and dry. The patient is oriented to person, place, and time. She has intact sensation and spontaneously moves all extremities, with significant pain noted in the left hip following any movement. Her pulse oximeter is 95% on room air. Postoperative hemoglobin is 9.8g/dL.

1. How would you describe the patient's type of pain?

2. How would you approach the ongoing assessment and management of the patient's pain?

3. What are the potential adverse effects of her pain treatment?

Terminology in musculoskeletal department

abduction 外展

adduction 内收

flexion 屈曲

anteflexion 前曲

dorsiflexion 背曲

ventriflexion 腹侧屈曲

rotation 旋转

pronation 旋前

supination 旋后

extension 伸直

forward bending 前弯

backward bending 后弯

lateral bending 侧弯

external rotation 外旋

internal rotation 内旋

limping 跛行

waddling gait 鸭步

kyphosis 脊柱后凸

lordosis 脊柱前凸

gibbus 驼背

posture scoliosis 姿势性侧凸

organic scoliosis 器质性侧凸

deformity 变形，畸形

retrograde degeneration 退行性变性

volar wrist cock-up 掌腕翘起

acropachy 杵状指

koilonychia 匙状甲

genu valgum 膝外翻

genu varum 膝内翻

flatfoot 扁平足

talipes equinus 马蹄足

talipes calcaneus 跟足畸形

talipes valgus 足外翻

pes cavus 高弓足

hemarthrosis 关节积血

arthrocentesis 关节穿刺术

straight leg raising test 直腿抬高试验

stenosing tenosynovitis 狭窄性腱鞘炎

tennis elbow 网球肘

shoulder-hand syndrome 肩手综合征

sicca syndrome 干燥综合征

carpal tunnel syndrome 腕管综合征

radial tunnel syndrome 桡管综合征

rheumatoid arthritis 类风湿性关节炎

synovitis 滑膜炎

ankylosing spondylitis 强直性脊柱炎

systemic lupus erythematosus(SLE) 系统性红斑狼疮

vasculitis 血管炎

takayasu arteritis 大动脉炎

hypersensitivity angitis 超敏性血管炎

enteropathic arthritis 肠病性关节炎

giant cell arteritis 巨细胞动脉炎

temporal arteritis 颞动脉炎

Behcet disease 白塞病

idiopathic inflammatory myositis 特发性炎症性肌病

polymyositis 多发性肌炎

dermatomyositis 皮肌炎

amyopathic dermatomyositis 无肌病性皮肌炎

juvenile dermatomyositis 幼年性皮肌炎

osteoarthritis 骨性关节炎

viral myositis 病毒性肌炎

relapsing polychondritis 复发性多发性软骨炎

hypertrophic osteoarthropathy 肥大性骨关节病

vasculitis 脉管炎

gout 痛风

Chapter 8

Endocrine System

Section A   Focus Listening

Conversation

Listen to the dialogue and fill in the blanks with proper words.

D=doctor P=patient

D: Ms. Liu, what seems to be the problem?

P: Dr. Cai, I had badly and profuse _____ in the last 2 months.

D: Have you had these problems before?

P: No.

D: Do you remember whether there is anything special bringing on these problems?

P: It's hard to say because it is a private event.

D: Don't worry. I'd like to find out what causes your problems. I'll keep it secret if etiology involved your privacy.

P: Um... My boyfriend broke up with me about two months ago. I hardly accept it. Since then, I have been in _____ condition for a long time.

D: Do you have any other symptoms?

P: I have shortness of breath and choking sensation in the chest sometimes.

D: I'd like to order ECG for you.

P: OK.

About half an hour, the patient came back with ECG results.

D: Let me see. The ECG shows that you have tachycardia and arrhythmia (premature atrial contraction). Does any your family member have heart diseases?

P: No.

D: I need to examine you first. Would you mind lifting up your shirt?

P: OK.

D: Um, the grade I _____ is heard with accentuated first heart sound. And would you please roll up your sleeves? I need to take your blood pressure.

P: What about my blood pressure?

D: 140 over 75, the widened pulse pressure presents. Please put your wrist on the table.

P: Is it serious?

D: I need more information to assess the condition. Oh, water hammer pulse presents, your skin is moist and warm. Have you found any weight loss, heat intolerance or fatigue?

P: Yes, I had a low-grade fever.

D: What's your appetite been like?

P: Eat like a horse but I still feel hungry at times, and I find I have been much slender than used to be.

D: Polyphagia, and what about your bowels, any problem?

P: Frequent bowel movement with undigested food.

D: Do you sleep well?

P: No, I have difficulty in falling asleep with restlessness and _____, my colleague told me I was sensitive and talkative in the last 2 months. What's more, I can't focus on my work and have poor memory.

D: What about your menstruation?

P: Scanty.

D: Let me examine you again. Now, swallow please. OK, I'll put my stethoscope to examine further. Um..., some continuous systolic murmur. Can you close your eyes? Yeah. OK, open them.

P: Doctor, what's wrong with me?

D: The stare and proptosis, also called as exophthalmos, presents. I'm going to order some tests for you, and I will see you again in one week, then I can make an exact _____ after get the results. I highly suspect that you had hyperthyroidism at the moment.

A few days later.

D: The value of your plasma TSH（Thyroid-stimulating hormone）is 0.06 μU/mL and the T3 resin-uptake ratio of 3 hour is 42%, which indicates that you have hyperthyroidism.

P: Is there anything that can be done about it?

D: I'll prescribe some medications for you. Attention please, the medications should be taken for about 1 to 2 years.

New Words & Expressions

interphalangeal 近端指间的

phalangeal 指骨的

anemia 贫血

rheumatoid arthritis 类风湿性关节炎

erythrocyte 红细胞

sedimentation 沉降

synovitis 滑膜炎

radiograph X 光照片

methotrexate 甲氨蝶呤

Passage

Answer the questions after listening to the passage.

1. Which of the following best describes the term Hirsutism?

A. Excess hair on the head.

B. Hair loss.

C. Excess hair on the face and neck.

D. Both A and B.

2. What is the most common cause of Cushing's syndrome?

A. Pituitary adenoma.

B. Adrenal tumor.

C. ACTC secreting ectopic tumors.

D. All of the above.

3. Which one of the following treatment method(s) is/are suitable for Cushing's Disease?

A. Surgery.

B. Radiotherapy.

C. Chemotherapy.

D. Both A and B.

4. Which one of the following hormone level is increased in Cushing's disease?

A. Insulin.

B. Thyroxine.

C. Cortisol.

D. Prolactin.

5. Which one of the following is NOT true regarding Cushing's disease?

A. Presence of moon face.

B. Presence of Buffalo hump.

C. Hirsutism.

D. Stunted growth.

Section B   Reading Comprehension

Text

A 13-year-old girl presents to the emergency department (ED) with 2 months of worsening shortness of breath, malaise, fever, and loose stools. She traveled to Mexico approximately 10 weeks ago. After her trip, she had non-bloody, frequent, loose stools for 2 weeks, then began having general malaise, with intermittent fevers every 2–3 weeks and dyspnea upon exertion. She reported sporadic shakiness, dizziness, diaphoresis, and tachycardia at rest. She also developed intermittent "burning" head pain and recurrence of loose stools.

She was evaluated by her primary care physician for dyspnea and was prescribed an albuterol inhaler, which had no effect. She had unremarkable pulmonary function testing and chest radiography findings. Inhaled ipratropium, intranasal fluticasone, and omeprazole had no effect. Allergy and otolaryngology specialists believed that her shortness of breath was secondary to vocal cord dysfunction.

Two weeks before her ED presentation, the patient experienced daily fevers for 1 week, with continued loose stools. Her pediatrician performed stool tests for Salmonella, Shigella, Campylobacter, and Clostridium difficile, which were all negative. No growth on blood and urine cultures was noted, Epstein-Barr serology was negative, and a tuberculin skin test was nonreactive.

The patient was started on amoxicillin for 10 days for presumed sinusitis. Her fever stopped on the 2nd day of antibiotics but returned, with a temperature as high as 103 °F on the 8th day of antibiotics, 3 days before her ED presentation. She continued to have up to four loose stools per day. Her headache became more severe and began to awaken her from sleep. She denied upper respiratory infection (URI) symptoms, cough, rash, night sweats, or persistent weight loss. She presented to the ED owing to worsening symptoms and persistent fevers.

Her family history is significant for a paternal grandmother with a rheumatologic disorder and a father with a resected thyroid mass; the etiology of both is unknown. Her social history is unremarkable, other than her recent travel to Mexico and exposure to a dog at home.

Physical Examination and Workup

Upon physical examination, the patient's temperature is 98.2 °F, blood pressure is 133/81 mmHg, heart rate is 145 beats/min, respiratory rate is 36 breaths/min, oxygen saturation is 100% in room air, and weight is 71.65 lb (32nd percentile). She appears nontoxic. Her head and neck examination is unremarkable, other than tenderness of the bilateral temporal areas. She is tachycardic, with normal S1 and S2 sounds and no murmurs. She is tachypneic, with clear lungs throughout and no accessory muscle use. Mild generalized abdominal and chest tenderness are present, with a soft abdomen and no guarding or rebound.

Preliminary laboratory findings are notable for a white blood cell count of 16,200/μL, hemoglobin level of 10.9 g/dL, platelet count of 309,000/μL, erythrocyte sedimentation rate of 23 mm/h, and C-reactive protein level of 3.7 mg/dL. Her electrolyte and liver enzyme findings are unremarkable. Blood culture results are pending, and urinalysis is negative. She is admitted for further evaluation of her unexplained fever.

The next morning, the patient develops a fever (100.8℉), with persistent resting tachycardia (142 beats/min) and tachypnea, even in absence of fever. She has abdominal pain, loose stool, and an episode of vomiting. She continues to have headache, which awakens her from sleep. Upon examination, she has new-onset disorientation, with word-finding difficulty.

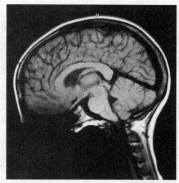

Figure 5 Image of brain MRI

A brain MRI is obtained, it was substantially limited by artifact from the patient's braces but otherwise revealed no acute intracranial abnormality (Figure 5).

Lumbar puncture is performed, and initial cerebrospinal fluid studies are negative, including cell count, differential, and Gram stain. Pediatric rheumatology and infectious disease specialists are consulted.

New Words & Expressions

sporadic [spə'rædɪk] *a.* happening fairly often, but not regularly 不时发生的，零星的

albuterol [æl'bju:tə,rɔ:l] *n.* 沙丁胺醇

intranasal [ˌɪntrə'neɪzəl] *a.* 鼻内的

otolaryngology ['əʊtəʊraɪnəʊlærɪŋ'gɒlədʒɪ] *n.* the ranch of medicine concerned with the ear, nose, and throat and their diseases 耳鼻喉医学

difficile [di:fɪ'si:l] *a.* hard, difficult（法）困难的；难相处的；固执的

sinusitis [ˌsaɪnə'saɪtɪs] *n.* a condition in which your sinuses swell up and become painful（鼻）窦炎

resect [rɪ'sekt] *v.* to cut out part of (a bone, an organ, or other structure or part) 切除（骨头、器官或其他组织的部分）

thyroid ['θaɪrɔɪd] *n.* an organ located near the base of the neck 甲状腺

etiology [ˌi:tɪ'ɒlədʒɪ] *n.* the cause of a disease or the scientific study of this ［病理］病因学；［基医］病原学；致病源

sedimentation [ˌsedɪmen'teɪʃ(ə)n] *n.* the natural process by which small pieces of rock, earth etc settle at the bottom of the sea etc and form a solid layer 沉积（作用）

pend [pend] *v.* to await judgment or settlement 等候判定或决定

new-onset *a.* 新发病的，初发病的

artifact ['ɑ:tɪfækt] *n.* a man-made object taken as a whole 人工制品；手工艺品

intracranial [ˌɪntrə'kreɪnɪəl] *a.* within the skull 颅内的

cerebrospinal [ˌserɪbrəʊ'spaɪnəl] *a.* of or relating to the brain and spinal cord 脑脊髓的

rheumatology [ˌru:mə'tɒlədʒɪ] *n.* the branch of medicine dealing with the study and treatment of pathologies of the muscles or tendons or joints 风湿病学

Exercise

Decide whether the following statements are true (T) or false (F) according to the passage.

_____1. The patient traveled to Mexico approximately 10 weeks ago, after her trip, she had non-bloody, frequent, tight stools for 3 weeks.

_____2. The girl had ordinary pulmonary function testing and chest radiography findings.

_____3. The patient's pediatrician got stool studies for Salmonella, Shigella, Campylobacter, and Clostridium difficile two weeks before her ED presentation, some of which were negative.

_____4. The girl's grandmother had a rheumatologic disorder and her father had a thyroid mass which was cut later.

_____5. In the next morning the patient had abdominal pain, loose stool, an episode of vomiting and continued to have headache.

Answer the following questions according to the passage.

1. What symptoms did the patient have when she presented to the emergency department?

_____

2. What were the results of the patient's stool studies 2 weeks before her ED presentation?

_____

3. What are her preliminary laboratory findings?

_____

Use the appropriate form of the words or phrases in the box to complete the following sentences.

new-onset	sporadic	artifact	sinusitis	pend
afebrile	thyroid	tachypnea	saturation	intracranial
cerebrospinal	resect	otolaryngology		

1. The patient presents to the emergency department within the first week of life in severe distress, including hypoxia, _____, and hypotension.

2. It's because we have these performers up there that are reading this blueprint and everyone is listening, basically to see how accurately they can reproduce, revivify this

artistic _____.

3. We also know Vitamin D activates and deactivates enzymes in the brain and the _____ fluid that are involved in neurotransmitter synthesis and never growth.

4. The patient is hospitalized with severe sepsis who experiences_____ atrial fibrillation and has an associated increased risk of in-hospital stroke and death, according to a study appearing in JAMA.

5. First, we need to identify more robust methods to predict the individual risk of ischemic stroke and bleeding — especially _____ hemorrhage.

6. The 1968 pandemic began relatively mild, with _____ cases prior to the first wave, and remained mild in its second wave in most, but not all countries.

7. If you're on time, you can _____ the tumor (depending on the site) without even needing to remove the pancreas or any other organ.

8. Located near the base of the neck, the _____ is a large endocrine gland that produces hormones that help control growth and metabolism.

9. Dr. Rice has also proposed studies to determine the most effective use — at what dosage, and for how long — of antibiotics for common infections like bronchitis and _____.

10. Emergent ophthalmologic and _____ consultation is warranted because surgical drainage may be necessary.

Translation

A. Translate the following expressions in to English.
1. 间歇性灼烧感头痛　　　　　　2. 声带功能异常
3. 结核菌素皮肤试验　　　　　　4. 红细胞沉降率
5. 腰椎穿刺　　　　　　　　　　6. 小儿风湿病学专家
7. 主治医师　　　　　　　　　　8. 双侧颞区的触痛

B. Translate the following sentences or expressions into Chinese.
1. A brain MRI is obtained; it was substantially limited by artifact from the patient's braces but otherwise revealed no acute intracranial abnormality.

2. She then began having general malaise, with intermittent fevers every 2-3 weeks and dyspnea upon exertion.

3. She denied upper respiratory infection (URI) symptoms, cough, rash, night sweats, or persistent weight loss.

4. Mild generalized abdominal and chest tenderness are present, with a soft abdomen and no guarding or rebound.

5. Her electrolyte and liver enzyme findings are unremarkable. Blood culture results are pending, and urinalysis is negative.

Section C　Vocabulary (Terminology)

1. 分泌 secrete

Combining form	Meaning	Terminology	Terminology meaning
crin/o	secrete	endocrinology	a branch of medicine concerned with the structure, function, and disorders of the endocrine glands 内分泌腺

2. 腺 gland

Combining form	Meaning	Terminology	Terminology meaning
aden/o	gland	lymphadenitis	inflammation of lymph nodes 淋巴腺炎

3. 肾上腺 adrenal glands

Combining form	Meaning	Terminology	Terminology meaning
adren/o	adrenal glands	adrenochrome	a red-colored mixture of quinones derived from epinephrine by oxidation 肾上腺色素，肾上腺素红
adrenal/o	adrenal glands	adrenalectomy	removal of adrenal gland 肾上腺切除术

4. 甲状腺 thyroid gland

Combining form	Meaning	Terminology	Terminology meaning
thyr/o	thyroid gland	thyrotropin	thyroid-stimulating hormone 促甲状腺素
thyroid/o		thyroiditis	inflammation of the thyroid gland 甲状腺炎

5. 性腺 sex glands, gonad

Combining form	Meaning	Terminology	Terminology meaning
gonad/o	sex gland (ovaries and testes)	gonadotropin	a gonadotropic hormone 促性腺激素

6. 垂体 pituitary gland, hypophysis

Combining form	Meaning	Terminology	Terminology meaning
pituitary/o	pituitary gland, hypophysis	hypopituitarism	deficient production of growth hormones by the pituitary gland 垂体功能减退症

7. 副甲状腺 parathyroid gland

Combining form	Meaning	Terminology	Terminology meaning
parathyroid/o	parathyroid gland	parathyroidectomy	partial or complete excision of the parathyroid glands 甲状腺切除术

8. 激素 hormone

Combining form	Meaning	Terminology	Terminology meaning
hormone/o	hormone	hormonal	of, relating to, or effected by hormones 激素的

9. 皮质，皮层 cortex, outer region

Combining form	Meaning	Terminology	Terminology meaning
cortic/o	cortex, outer region	corticosteroid	any of various adrenal-cortex steroids (as corticosterone, cortisone, and aldosterone) used medically especially as anti-inflammatory agents 皮质类固醇

10. 实质 solid structure

Combining form	Meaning	Terminology	Terminology meaning
ster/o	solid structure	steroid	any of various compounds containing a 17-carbon 4-ring system and including the sterols and numerous hormones (as anabolic steroids or corticosteroids) and glycosides 类固醇

11. 女性 female

Combining form	Meaning	Terminology	Terminology meaning
estr/o	female	estrogen	any of various natural steroids (as estradiol) that are formed from androgen precursors 雌激素

12. 男性 female

Combining form	Meaning	Terminology	Terminology meaning
andr/o	male	androgen	a male sex hormone 雄性激素

13. 胰岛素 insulin

Combining form	Meaning	Terminology	Terminology meaning
insulin/o	insulin	insulinase	enzyme relating to insulin 胰岛素酶

14. 乳，奶 milk

Combining form	Meaning	Terminology	Terminology meaning
lact/o	milk	prolactin	a protein hormone of the anterior lobe of the pituitary that induces lactation 催乳素
galact/o	milk	galactorrhea	a spontaneous flow of milk from the nipple 乳溢

15. 相同 sameness

Combining form	Meaning	Terminology	Terminology meaning
home/o	sameness	homeostasis	a relatively stable state of equilibrium or a tendency toward such a state between the different but interdependent elements or groups of elements of an organism, population, or group 体内平衡

16. 黏液 mucus

Combining form	Meaning	Terminology	Terminology meaning
myx/o	mucus	myxedema	severe hypothyroidism characterized by firm inelastic edema, dry skin and hair, and loss of mental and physical vigor 黏液水肿

17. 体 body

Combining form	Meaning	Terminology	Terminology meaning
somat/o	body	somatotropin	growth hormone 生长激素

18. 分娩，生产 childbirth

Combining form	Meaning	Terminology	Terminology meaning
toc/o	child birth	oxytocin	a pituitary octapeptide hormone $C_{43}H_{66}N_{12}O_{12}S_2$ that stimulates especially the contraction of uterine muscle and the secretion of milk 催产素

19. 毒，毒药，毒物 poison

Combining form	Meaning	Terminology	Terminology meaning
toxic/op	poison	thyrotoxicosis	excessive functional activity of the thyroid gland 甲状腺毒症

20. 钙 calcium

Combining form	Meaning	Terminology	Terminology meaning
calc/o	calcium	hypercalcemia	an excess of calcium in the blood 高钙血症

21. 钾 potassium

Combining form	Meaning	Terminology	Terminology meaning
kali	potassium	hypokalemia	a deficiency of potassium in the blood 低钾血症

22. 钠 sodium

Combining form	Meaning	Terminology	Terminology meaning
natr/o	sodium	hyponatremia	a deficiency of sodium in the blood 低钠血症

23. 生长 growing

Combining form	Meaning	Terminology	Terminology meaning
phys/o	growing	hypophysectomy	surgical removal of the pituitary gland 垂体切除术

24. 集合，召集，聚集 assemble, gather together

Combining form	Meaning	Terminology	Terminology meaning
-agon	assemble, gather together	glucagon	a protein hormone that is produced especially by the islets of Langerhans and that promotes an increase in the sugar content of the blood by increasing the rate of glycogen breakdown in the liver 胰高血糖激素

25. 物质 substance

Combining form	Meaning	Terminology	Terminology meaning
-in		adrenocorticotropin	a protein hormone of the anterior lobe of the pituitary gland that stimulates the adrenal cortex 促肾上腺皮质激素
-ine	substance	epinephrine	a colorless crystalline feebly basic sympathomimetic hormone $C_9H_{13}NO_3$ that is the principal blood-pressure raising hormone secreted by the adrenal medulla and is used medicinally especially as a heart stimulant 肾上腺素

26. 促进功能 stimulating the function of (to turn or act upon)

Combining form	Meaning	Terminology	Terminology meaning
-tropin	stimulating the function of (to turn or act on)	adrenocorticotropin	a protein hormone of the anterior lobe of the pituitary gland that stimulates the adrenal cortex 促肾上腺皮质激素

27. 尿的情况 urine condition

Combining form	Meaning	Terminology	Terminology meaning
-uria	urine condition	glycosuria	the presence in the urine of abnormal amounts of sugar 糖尿

28. 正常的，好的 good, normal

Combining form	Meaning	Terminology	Terminology meaning
eu-	good, normal	euthyroid	characterized by normal thyroid function 甲状腺功能正常的

29. 快速、敏捷 rapid, sharp, acid

Combining form	Meaning	Terminology	Terminology meaning
oxy-	rapid, sharp, acid	oxytocin	a pituitary octapeptide hormone $C_{43}H_{66}N_{12}O_{12}S_2$ that stimulates especially the contraction of uterine muscle and the secretion of milk 催产素

30. 渴 thirst

Combining form	Meaning	Terminology	Terminology meaning
dys/o	thirst	polydipsia	excessive or abnormal thirst 大渴

31. 三 three

Combining form	Meaning	Terminology	Terminology meaning
tri-	three	triodothyronine	an iodine-containing hormone $C_{15}H_{12}I_3NO_4$ that is an amino acid derived from thyroxine 三碘甲腺原氨酸 (T_3)

32. 四 four

Combining form	Meaning	Terminology	Terminology meaning
tetra-	four	tetraiodothyronine	四碘甲状腺原氨酸 (T₄)

Exercise for vocabulary

Match the following pathological conditions or terms with their meanings below.

gonadotropin	corticosteroid	glycagon	thyrotropin
adrenochrome	oxytocin	androgen	estrogen
homeostasis	adrenocorticotropin	prolactin	hypercalcemia
glycosuria	hypokalemia	somatotropin	endocrinology
tr Ⅱ odothyronine	lymphadenitis	myxedema	hyponatremia

_____1. Inflammation of lymph nodes.

_____2. A gonadotropic hormone.

_____3. A protein hormone that is produced especially by the islets of Langerhans and that promotes an increase in the sugar content of the blood by increasing the rate of glycogen breakdown in the liver.

_____4. A red-colored mixture of quinones derived from epinephrine by oxidation.

_____5. A relatively stable state of equilibrium or a tendency toward such a state between the different but interdependent elements or groups of elements of an organism, population, or group.

_____6. The presence in the urine of abnormal amounts of sugar.

_____7. A pituitary octapeptide hormone $C_{43}H_{66}N_{12}O_{12}S_2$ that stimulates especially the contraction of uterine muscle and the secretion of milk.

_____8. A protein hormone of the anterior lobe of the pituitary that induces lactation.

_____9. Any of various natural steroids (as estradiol) that are formed from androgen precursors, that are secreted chiefly by the ovaries, placenta, adipose tissue, and testes, and that stimulate the development of female secondary sex characteristics and promote the growth and maintenance of the female reproductive system, also: any of various synthetic or semisynthetic steroids (as ethinyl estradiol) that mimic the physiological effect of natural estrogens.

_____10. A protein hormone of the anterior lobe of the pituitary gland that stimulates the adrenal cortex.

_____11. Thyroid-stimulating hormone.

_____12. Any of various adrenal-cortex steroids (as corticosterone, cortisone, and aldosterone) used medically especially as anti-inflammatory agents.

_____13. An iodine-containing hormone $C_{15}H_{12}I_3NO_4$ that is an amino acid derived from thyroxine.

_____14. A branch of medicine concerned with the structure, function, and disorders of the endocrine glands.

_____15. Severe hypothyroidism characterized by firm inelastic edema, dry skin and hair, and loss of mental and physical vigor.

_____16. A deficiency of potassium in the blood.

_____17. A deficiency of sodium in the blood.

_____18. An excess of calcium in the blood.

_____19. A male sex hormone (as testosterone).

_____20. Produced by the anterior lobe of the pituitary gland, also called growth hormone.

Choose the term that best matches the meanings of the sentences.

1. Miss Wu, aged 28 and unmarried, presents your office complaining of palpitation, heat intolerance and profuse sweats for over 2 months. She stated that she had the history of asthma. On physical examination: exophthalmos, grade II enlargement of thyroid, systolic murmur heard on apex of both thyroids, heart rate 120 beats/min, T_3 3.2ng/mL, T_4 196μg/mL, T_3 resin-uptake ratio:3h 39%, 24h 92%. What's the most likely diagnosis?

　　A. Grave's disease.　　　　　　　　B. Tachycardia.
　　C. Simple goiter.　　　　　　　　　D. PAC/premature atrial contractions.

2. A 20-year-old unmarried female presented with palpitation, moist and warm skin and increased sweats over 3 months. On physical examination: grade II enlargement of thyroid, arteries sound heard on apex of the right thyroid. Which of following mostly can't present in the history taking and physical examination?

　　A. Fine resting finger tremor.　　　　B. Water hammer pulse.
　　C. Exophthalmos.　　　　　　　　　D. Menorrhagia.

3. A married female's facial feature gradually became "rough" in her late thirties and forties. At her age of 50, her children noticed her very large hands and recommended that she saw an endocrinologist, who diagnosed her chronically progressive conditions as_____?

　　A. hyperinsulinism　　　　　　　　B. gigantism
　　C. acromegaly　　　　　　　　　　D. hypothyroidism

4. A 48-year-old female presented with fatigue, menorrhagia and myalgia for more than 10 years and facial and periorbital edema over 2 weeks. She stated that she had cold

intolerance, poor memory, constipation and hoarseness. On physical examination: pallor complexion, depression, dry skin, heart rate 52 beats/min, and tendon reflex relaxation. What is the most likely diagnosis?

A. Hyperthyroidism.   B. Thyroiditis.

C. Hypothyroidism.   D. Cushing syndrome.

5. Mary noticed that she had gained weight recently and her face had a moon-like fullness with new heavy hair growth. Blood and urine test showed excessive secretion of adrenal glucocorticoids, CT scan of the abdomen revealed enlargement of both adrenal glands. Her doctor made the diagnosis of_____.

A. Grave's disease   B. Cushing syndrome

C. chronic adrenocortical hypofunction   D. primary aldosteronism

6. Phyllis was diagnosed with Gravis disease when her husband noticed her _____. Her eyes seemed to be bulging out of their sockets.

A. panhypopituitarism   B. hirsutism

C. exophthalmos   D. myocardial ischemia

7. Bobby was brought into the emergency room because he was found passed out in the kitchen. He had forgotten his insulin injection and developed _____.

A. Cushing disease   B. hyperparathyroidism

C. diabetic ketoacidosis   D. pseudobulbar palsy

8. Because her 1- hour test of blood sugar was slightly abnormal, Sema's obstetrician ordered a _____ to rule out gestational diabetes.

A. glucose tolerance test   B. thyroid function test

C. Pap smear   D. blood sugar

9. Helen had a primary brain tumor called a _____ adenoma. her entire endocrine system was disrupted, and her physician recommended surgery and radiation to help relieve her symptoms.

A. pituitary   B. thyroid   C. adrenal   D. dystonia

10. Grave's disease, as characterized by exophthalmos and stare, was diagnosed in a 51-year-old man. Examination revealed a history of nervousness, palpitation, weight loss, diarrhea, dyspnea on exertion, insomnia, heat intolerance, and fatigue. An ECG showed atrial fibrillation with a ventricular rate of about 180 beats per minute, which was treated with digoxin and propranolol. A chest x-ray film disclosed cardiomegaly. Thyroid function tests showed T4 and T3 levels to be elevated, and a thyroid scan showed diffuse enlargement of the gland. The patient was treated with radioactive iodine and is now euthyroid. The exophthalmos has not resolved, Symptoms of Grave's disease are:

A. bulging eyeballs   B. difficult breathing on exertion

C. acromegaly   D. A and B

Section D   Writing

Review of system

对于许多医学生而言，系统回顾部分 (review of system, ROS) 好比是一个沼泽地，很容易在其中迷失。把它想象成你正在建造的阁楼，阁楼里可以放置一些你特别感兴趣，同时又非常重要的东西，但并不是一些显然应该放在别处的东西也可以放在此处的。简而言之，系统回顾就是从头到脚各个系统的详细罗列，包括任何与现在主诉症状无直接关系，但对进一步评估有用的东西。这是对健康的真实描述，其重要性次于现病史。任何与当前临床表现相关的阳性结果和阴性结果，都应归属于现病史，而非系统回顾。系统回顾是描述一些最近发生的或尚处于活动期的疾病，而非很久以前发生的疾病。

Example 1

Review of Systems (ROS):

Head: Denies recent trauma, occasional frontal headaches with no associated symptoms of sinus drainage. Jaw pain, visual changes, nausea, vomiting, or aura. Headache relieved by Tylenol.

Eyes: Denies blurring, double version, flashes/floaters, eye pain, needs reading glasses.

Ears: Denies hearing loss, tinnitus, or ear pain.

Nose: Denies decreased smell, rhinorrhea, epistaxis.

Throat: Denies sore throat, odynophagia/dysphagia, abnormal taste, halitosis.

Neck: Denies stiffness.

Palm: See HPI.

CV: See HPI, no palpitation, orthopnea, paroxysmal nocturnal dyspnea, or edema but does feel occasional "skipped beats" that last only a second and occur 2~3x/week. Denies Raynaud's.

GI: See HPI, denies bloating, cramping, change in stool color/quality, or bright red blood per rectum. Positive heartburn exacerbated by alcohol and relieved usually by milk or antacids. Besides, midepigastric gnawing pain increased after eating over last weeks, again, mildly improved by antacids.

GU: Denies dysuria, penile discharge, erectile or ejaculatory dysfunction.

Musculoskeletal: No joint pain except R knee from old sports injury. Denies swelling of joints and muscular pain/weakness.

Derm: See HPI.

Endocrine: Denies heat /cold intolerance, no recent changes in hat/glove size.

Psych: Denies depressed mood, sleep difficulties, or anxiety. States history of seeing bugs crawling on the wall when he stopped drinking alcohol for a few days, he did note one episode about 6 weeks ago when he stopped drinking alcohol for a few days and began seeing bugs crawling on the walls that on one else saw. But the phenomenon stopped when he resumed drinking.

从上例我们可以看出这是用简洁的若干短句来完成系统的写作，要求重点突出，事实清楚。我们再看一个实例：

Example 2

Review of systems (ROS):

General/constitutional: Pt. denies fever/chills, fatigue, weakness, weight changes greater than ten pounds, appetite changes, temperature intolerance, or sleep problems.

HEENT: Denies eye pain, redness, loss of vision, double or blurred vision, flashing lights or spots, dryness, the feeling of a foreign object in the eye. Uses soft contact lenses during the day and glasses at night for correction of nearsightedness. Denies tinnitus, hearing loss, uses of hearing aids. Denies history of nose bleeds, dry sinuses, loss of sense of smell, sore tongue, bleeding gums, mouth sores, loss of sense of taste, dry mouth, dentures, mouth sores, frequent sore throats, hoarseness or feeling of need to clear the throat. Denies acid or bitter fluid in the mouth or throat upon awakening. Denies difficult or painful swallowing. States history of chronic sinusitis and post nasal drip.

Cardiovascular: Denies chest pain, irregular heartbeats, sudden changes in heartbeat or palpitation, difficulty breathing at night, heart murmurs, high blood pressure, edema, cramps in legs with walking, pain in feet or toes at night or varicose veins, syncope, dyspnea.

Respiratory: Denies chronic dry cough, hemoptysis, coughing up mucus/sputum production, waking at night coughing or choking, repeated pneumonias, night sweats, wheezing with or without exercise, respiratory chest pain, dyspnea on exertion. Notes positive history of asthma.

Gastrointestinal: Denies Nausea, vomiting, vomiting blood or coffee ground-like emesis, heartburn, regurgitation, frequent belching, dysphagia, retrosternal burning, abdominal/rectal pain, stomach pain relieved by food, yellow jaundice(skin or eyes), diarrhea, constipation, excessive gas, blood in the stools, black tarry stools, hemorrhoids, stool incontinence.

Genitourinary: Denies difficulty urinating, pain or burning with urination, blood in the urine, cloudy or smoky urine, urinary frequency, nocturia, urinary incontinence, kidney stones, rash or ulcers in the genital area, sexual dysfunction, or sexually transmitted diseases. Denies vaginal discharge; s/p hysterectomy 5 years ago.

Musculoskeletal: Denies bilateral UE or LE cramps, joint or muscle pain, muscle weakness/tenderness, joint edema; neck or back pain. History of right inversion ankle sprain in 2009.

Integumentary & Breasts: Denies changes in skin/air, easy bruising, skin redness, rash, hives sensitivity to sun exposure, tightness, nodules or bumps. Denies hair loss, color changes in the hands or feet with cold, persistent lesion, changes in mole(s), fingernail changes; breast lumps, pain or nipple discharge.

Neurological: Denies headache, dizziness, muscle spasm, loss of consciousness, sensitivity or pain in the hands and feet, memory loss, balance or walking difficulties, diplopia.

Psychiatric: Denies depression, thoughts of suicide, hearing voices without the presence of other people in the room/hallucinating, usual eating habits, obsessive/compulsive habits, manic/depressed moods, excessive anxiety, problems with memory, problems with concentration, problems with thinking, previous abuse by others.

Endocrine: Denies intolerance to hot or cold temperature, flushing, increased thirst, increased salt intake. Decreased sexual desire. States history of adrenal insufficiency and hypothyroidism.

Hematological/lymphatic: Denies anemia, bleeding tendency, clotting tendency.

Allergic/immunologic: States history or rhinitis, received allergen immunotherapy by injection from age of 4. Denies skin sensitivity, latex allergies or sensitivity.

Physical examination(PE)

系统性地进行体格检查，如一般情况、生命体征、头、眼、耳、鼻、喉、颈、肺、心脏、乳腺、腹部、直肠、生殖器、四肢、肌肉骨骼、神经系统。

在书写体格检查时，应该通过体格检查上的结果来进一步支持或否定前面提出的鉴别诊断。书写体格检查可以用完整的句子，也可以用短句。

Example

General: The patient appears cachectic, diaphoretic, in obvious respiratory distress, anxious, and older than his stated age.

Vitals: T=37.2℃ HR=144 (irr/irr-weak), BP=98/54 mmHg, RR=28 and labored.

Skin: moist without rashes, no tenting

HEENT (head, eyes, ears, nose, throat): sclera anicteric, PERRL (pupils equal, round, and reactive to light) bilaterally. Swing test not performed. Funduscopic exam: normal disk and vessels bilaterally, but exam limited by the patient's difficulty keeping eyes still. Tympanic membranes pearly and shows a cone of light bilaterally with normal external canals. The OP (oropharynx) was moist with mind erythema of the tonsillar pillars without exudates or petechiae. Dentition normal.

Neck: Supple with soft Nt (non-tender) cervical LAN (lymphadenopathy) in the anterior cervical chain. There was no supraclavicular lymphadenopathy noted. The thyroid was normal.

Pulmonary: Lung expansion is symmetric bilaterally. Auscultation reveals rales bilaterally about 2/3 of the way up the back. There is egophony with decreased fremitus at both bases. No wheezes or rhonchi noted. There is dullness to percussion at the R>L base.

Cor or CV (cardiovascular): The PMI (point of maximal impulse) was 4–5cm in size, diffuse, and laterally displaced to the anterior axillary line. The heart beating was tachycardic and irregular with an S1, S2, and S3-difficult to hear with loud breathing. There was no murmur. The carotids were 1+ bilaterally without bruits and the JVP (jugular venous pressure) was estimated at 10 cm.

Abd (abdomen): The abdomen revealed normal active bowel sounds. It was ND (non-distended) but minimally tender in the RUQ (right upper quadrant). There was rebound or guarding. The liver was palpated 3 finger-breadths below the right costal margin at the midclavicular line and was smooth in texture. The spleen was not palpable.

Rectal: Exam revealed guaiac-negative brown stool with normal tone and prostate exam.

Pelvic/GU: Normal circumcised phallus with no masses or discharges and normally descended testicles.

Extremities: There was no evidence of clubbing or cyanosis. He had 2+ pitting of his LE (lower extremities) to the knees. Bilateral radial, brachial, and femoral pulses were 2+. The dorsalis pedis and anterior tibial pulse were difficult to palpate due to edema. There was a femoral, axillary, or epitrochlear lymphadenopathy noted.

Musculoskeletal: There was full ranges of motion of all joints in the upper and lower extremities except right hip flexion which was only 40° limited by the patient's complaints of pain in the popliteal area. There was evidence of thickening of the MCP (metacarpophalangeal) joints on all fingers of both hands. None was warm, red or tender. There was no evidence of joints effusions.

Neurologic: cervical nerves (CN)

Ⅰ - not tested.

Ⅱ - able to read newspaper print with reading glasses one eye at a time.

Ⅲ - Ⅳ and Ⅵ - extraocular movement intact.

Ⅴ - facial light touch sensation normal.

Ⅶ - forehead wrinkles normally, no loss of facial folds.

Ⅷ - patient able to hear whispers bilaterally at 3 inches.

Ⅸ , Ⅹ - palate raises symmetrically, gag reflex intact.

Ⅺ - shoulder shrug strong bilaterally.

Ⅻ - tongue protrudes without deviation.

Sensory: Light touching, pin prick, and proprioceptive sensation on the hands and feet were normal.

Motor: Tone seems normal throughout, but muscles appear diffusely atrophied.

Coordination: Finger-nose-finger, heel-to-shin, fine finger movements and rapid alternating movement were all normal. Romberg testing was not performed.

Gait: Not tested due to breathlessness.

Mental status: Due to breathlessness, formal mental status testing was deferred. He was, however, alert and oriented to person, place and date.

Section E   Spoken English

Role play

Directions: A patient had a cold when she went out for dinner with some friends. The weather was extremely bad recently. So, when she came back, she had sneezing, cold aversion etc. Her husband went to clinic for help. 2 students are selected to demonstrate the conversation, one plays the role of doctor, the other of patient.

Discussion

Directions: Work in groups and discuss with your partners, then answer the following questions with detailed analysis.

A 55-year-old African American female presents to clinic as a new patient. She has not seen a physician in many years and would like a general health checkup. The patient is not treated for any chronic health problems. However, her mother had Type 2 diabetes, and she would like to be screened.

Physical examination is unremarkable except for weight of 180 lb(81.8 kg; height 165 cm, BMI 30.3 kg/m^2). The patient has multiple risk factors for type 2 diabetes including age, ethnicity, and family history that justify screening. Since the patient is not fasting, hemoglobin Alc (HbAlc)is measured and found to be elevated at 6.8%. Morning fasting plasma glucose is 145 mg/dL.

The patient returns to the office to discuss management of her newly diagnosed Type 2 diabetes. She is started on metformin and titrated to 1000 mg twice daily without side effects. She also modifies her diet and starts an exercise program. Three months later, capillary blood glucose measurements are consistently below 130 mg/dL, and HbAlc improves to 6.0%. Four years later, HbAlc increases steadily to 7.5% despite compliance with diet, exercise, and metformin. Dilated fundoscopy and foot examination are unremarkable, and urine albumin/Cr ratio remains below 30 mg/g.

Initially, HbAlc improves with the addition of glimepiride to metformin. Exenatide is then started 18 months later due to worsening glycemic control. Two years later, the patient returns to discuss treatment options. Despite taking maximal effective doses of metformin (1000 mg BID), glimepiride (8 mg QD), and exenatide (10 µg BID), HbAlc is 8.5%. Fasting glucose measurements fall mostly in the range of 140 to 180 mg/dL, and glucose measurements during the day increase steadily and are often more than 200 mg/dL.

1. Who should be screened for Type 2 diabetes mellitus?

2. How is Type 2 diabetes initially managed?

3. What regular screening is necessary for Type 2 diabetes patients?

4. What additional therapies can be added if metformin monotherapy is ineffective?

5. What is the next step in management for patients with progressively worsening glycemic control despite multiple oral medications or glucagon-like peptide-1(GLP-1) analog therapy?

Terminology in endocrine department

T$_3$ resin-uptake ratio 吸碘率

simple goiter 单纯性甲状腺瘤

growth hormone deficiency dwarfism 生长激素缺乏性侏儒症

hypopituitarism 垂体功能减退症

gigantism 巨人症

acromegaly 肢端肥大症

diabetes insipidus 尿崩症

arginine vasopressin 精氨酸加压素

antidiuretic hormone 抗利尿激素

neurophysin 神经垂体激素运载蛋白

syndrome of inappropriate antidiuretic hormone secretion 抗利尿激素分泌失调综合征

hyperthyroidism 甲状腺功能亢进症

Grave's disease Grave's 病

Hypothyroidism 甲状腺功能减退症

thyroiditis 甲状腺炎

subacute thyroiditis 亚急性甲状腺炎

chronic lymphocytic thyroiditis 慢性淋巴细胞性甲状腺炎

Cushing syndrome 库欣综合征

primary aldosteronism 原发性醛固酮增多症

chronic adrenocortical hypofunction 慢性肾上腺皮质功能减退症

pheochromocytoma 嗜铬细胞瘤

hyperparathyroidism 甲状旁腺功能亢进症

hypoparathyroidism 甲状旁腺功能减退症

thyroxine 甲状腺素

triiodothyronine 三碘甲状腺原氨酸

tetraiodothyronine 四碘甲状腺原氨酸

free triiodothyronine 游离三碘甲状腺原氨酸

thyroid hormone insensitivity syndrome 甲状腺不敏感综合征

reverse triiodothyronine 反三碘甲状腺原氨酸

thyroxine-binding globulin 甲状腺素结合球蛋白

parathyroid hormone 甲状旁腺素

parathormone 甲状旁腺素

calcitonin 降钙素

17-hydroxycorticosteroid 17- 羟皮质类固醇

17-ketosteroid 17- 酮皮质类固醇

cortisol 皮质醇

cortisol binding globulin 皮质醇结合蛋白

aldosterone 醛固酮

catecholamines 儿茶酚胺

testosterone 睾酮

estradiol 雌二醇

progesterone 黄体酮

thyroid stimulating hormone 促甲状腺激素

thyrotropin releasing hormone 促甲状腺激素释放激素

somatostatin 生长抑素

corticotropic hormone releasing hormone 促肾上腺皮质激素释放激素

growth hormone 生长激素

growth hormone releasing hormone 生长激素释放激素

growth hormone releasing inhibitory hormone 生长激素释放激素抑制激素

antidiuretic hormone 抗利尿激素

vasopressin 血管升压素

gonadotropic hormone（gonadotropin）促性腺激素

prolactin 催乳素

oxytocin 催产素

proptosis 眼球突出（症）

exophthalmos 眼球突出（症）

water hammer pulse 水冲脉

Chapter 9

Blood System

Section A   Focus Listening

Conversation

Listen to the dialogue and fill in the blanks with proper words.

M=mother D=doctor P=patient

M: Doctor, my daughter is running a temperature!

D: What's your daughter's temperature?

M: It's 37.8℃ when the nurse _____ for my daughter.

D: Any other symptoms?

M: Pain over the major the joints.

D: Does she have sneezing, running nose and sore throat?

M: Not yet.

D: How old is your daughter?

P: 16.

D: Do you have dizziness, fatigue _____, tinnitus and short breath after exertion since your face is pallor?

P: Yes. It's getting worse now.

D: When did your _____ start?

P: It began when I was at the age of 12.

D: And is your period regular?

P: No, my period has been getting much heavier recently.

D: Do you often bruise on your body?

P: Yes, I do.

D: Do your gums bleed when you brush your teeth?

P: Yes, quite a lot.

D: I'd like to order a CBC test and come back.

P: OK.

About 10 minutes later the patient and her mother came back with results.

D: Oh, your CBC test shows the WBC 36×10^9/L, I'd like to examine you first.

P: OK.

D: Is any problem with your eyes?

P: No.

D: You see there are 3 supraclavicular enlarged _____ nodes, does it hurt when I press on it?

P: No.

D: Is it painful when I press the lower end of breastbone?

P: Yes, it hurts. Doctor, what's wrong with me?

D: All the symptoms and signs are indicative that you may have acute leukemia, but I can't make the diagnosis until the results of examination of cell and _____ cell is presented.

M: Acute leukemia, My God. What can I do now?

D: You need to finish the examination I ordered for you; we'll take immediately shortly after the results are presented.

New Words & Expressions

menarche（月经）初潮　　　　　　　supraclavicular 锁骨上的

CBC 全血细胞　　　　　　　　　　　leukemia 白血病

Passage

Answer the questions after listening to the passage.

1. Which of the blood cells is affected in Leukemia?

A. Red blood cells.　　　　　　　　　B. White blood cells.

C. Platelets.　　　　　　　　　　　　D. All of the above.

2. What are the classical symptoms of Leukemia?

A. Sudden loss of weight.　　　　　　B. Loss of appetite.

C. Frequent infections.　　　　　　　D. All of the above.

3. Which of the following treatment method(s) is/are suitable for Leukemia?

A. Bone marrow transplant.　　　　　B. Surgery.

C. Chemotherapy.　　　　　　　　　D. Both A and C.

4. Which of the following is NOT the risk factor for Leukemia?

A. Exposure to benzene.　　　　　　　B. Smoking.

C. Alcohol consumption.　　　　　　　D. Radiation exposure.

5. In Leukemia the tendency of frequent infections are due to_____?

A. Abnormal blood cells.　　　　　　　B. Abnormal white blood cells.

C. Abnormal platelets.　　　　　　　　D. None of the above.

Section B　Reading Comprehension

Text

A 6-year-old South Asian girl presented in October 2013 with generalized bruises, undocumented fever, and eczematous rashes of 1 month's duration. She had had six or seven episodes of loose stools per day for 3 months accompanied by loss of appetite. She was a known asthmatic. Her family history was unknown as she was an adopted child. Her foster parents did not notice any food allergens. On examination, she was short with a height of 98 cm (< 5th percentile) and weight of 13.5 kg (< 5th percentile). There was pallor, multiple generalized petechiae, and eczematous patches on upper back and behind her ears with typical Fanconi facies including microcephaly and microphthalmia. A systemic examination was normal and no lymphadenopathy was appreciated.

Investigations revealed hemoglobin of 9.0g/dL, platelet count of 67×10^9/L, and mean corpuscular volume (MCV) and mean corpuscular hemoglobin (MCH) of 75.3 fl and 24.2 pg, respectively with no atypical cells. A liver function test (LFT), renal function test (RFT), urine examination, and coagulation profile were normal and blood culture was sterile. Ultrasonography of her abdomen and portal venous Doppler were normal. Antinuclear antibodies (ANA) titer was negative. Mitomycin C was used to detect chromosomal breakages to rule out Fanconi anemia and results were negative with 0.58 breaks/cell. Investigations for malabsorption revealed gamma A immunoglobulin (IgA) tissue transglutaminase levels to be 370 IU/mL (normal < 12 IU/mL), anti-gliadin antibodies to be 140 IU/mL (normal < 12 IU/mL), but normal thyroid profile. A jejunal biopsy showed complete villous atrophy with increased intraepithelial lymphocytes consistent with diagnosis of CD. She was managed with antibiotics, packed red cells, and platelet support and was put on a gluten-free diet. She was supplemented with multivitamins, vitamin C, and iron. She was discharged on day 17 of hospital stay with hemoglobin of 7.9 g/L, total leukocyte count of 2.5×10^9/L, and platelet count of 46×10^9/L. A bone marrow biopsy was advised. The household was noncompliant to follow ups with yearly follow ups showing varying platelet levels from $34 \times 10^9/L$ to $124 \times 10^9/L$.

The child presented in October 2016 with nonproductive cough, fever, respiratory distress for 2 months, and a history of recurrent infections over the past year. Her hemoglobin was 7.5 g/L, total leukocyte count of $3.5 \times 10^9/L$, and platelet count of $80 \times 10^9/L$. High-resolution computed tomography (HRCT) was suggestive of a lung abscess. Lung culture revealed Pseudomonas aeruginosa. GeneXpert, galactomannan, and β-d-glucan (BDG) antibodies were negative. She was managed symptomatically with blood transfusions and platelet support. A bone marrow trephine biopsy was done after consent that revealed hypocellular bone marrow with decreased lymphoid cells, plasma cells, erythroid and myeloid precursors with occasional megakaryocytes. We advised that the child have a bone marrow transplantation but the family refused due to financial constraints. The parents were counseled about the nature of the disease and treatment modalities. She is managed with packed red cells, platelet support, and a gluten-free diet; she showed an increasing trend in platelet count on last follow up.

Table 1 shows a timeline for our patient's past medical history and follow-up visits as well as interventions.

Table 1. Timeline of patient's medical history

Past medical history

A 6-year-old girl with history of bruising and fever for 1 month and loose stools for 3 months. She was a known asthmatic. Her family history was unknown as she was an adopted child

	Hospital/out-patient visits	Diagnostic tests	Interventions
October 2013	Presented with bruises, undocumented fever, and eczematous rashes for 1 month. Petechiae all over the body. Loose stools daily for 3 months with loss of appetite	Hb 9.0 g/dL, platelet 67 × $10^9/L$, MCV 75.3 fl, MCH 24.2 pg. Normal LFT, RFT, urine examination, and coagulation profile. Blood culture was sterile. ANA titer was negative. Chromosomal breakages was negative with 0.58 breaks/cell, IgA TTG 370 IU/mL, anti-gliadin antibodies 140 IU/mL. Jejunal biopsy-complete villous atrophy with increased intraepithelial lymphocytes	Antibiotics, packed red cells, and platelet support given. Put on a gluten-free diet, supplemented with multivitamins, vitamin C, and iron. She was discharged on day 17 of hospital stay with Hb 7.9g/L, TLC 2.5 × $10^9/L$, platelet count of 46 × $10^9/L$, and gluten-free diet. Bone marrow biopsy was advised
	Noncompliant with yearly follow ups	Varying platelet levels from 34 × $10^9/L$ to 124 × $10^9/L$	Gluten-free diet
October 2016	Nonproductive cough, fever, respiratory distress for 2 months. History of recurrent infections over the year	Lung abscess and a cavitary lesion seen on HRCT. Lung culture revealed Pseudomonas aeruginosa. GeneXpert, galactomannan, and BDG antibodies were negative. A bone marrow trephine biopsy revealed hypocellular bone marrow	She is planned for bone marrow transplantation. Parents were counseled about the disease and treatment. Managed with packed red cells, platelet support, and a gluten-free diet. She showed an increasing trend in platelet count

ANA antinuclear antibodies, *BDG* β-d-glucan, *Hb* hemoglobin, *HRCT* high-resolution computed tomography, *LFT* liver function test *MCH* mean corpuscular hemoglobin, *MCV* mean corpuscular volume, *RFT* renal function test, *TLC* total leukocyte count, *TTG* tissue transglutaminase.

New Words & Expressions

eczematous [ekˈsemətəs] *a.* 湿疹的

asthmatic [æsˈmætɪk] *n.* a person suffering from asthma 气喘患者，哮喘患者

pallor [ˈpælə] *n.* unnatural lack of color in the skin (as from bruising or sickness or emotional distress) 苍白；青白；灰白

microcephaly [ˌmaɪkrouˈsefəli] *n.* an abnormally small head and underdeveloped brain 小头畸形

microphthalmia [maɪkrəfˈθælmɪə] *n.* 小眼畸形

lymphadenopathy [ˈlɪmˌfædənˈɔpəθi] *n.* chronic abnormal enlargement of the lymph nodes (usually associated with disease) 淋巴结病

corpuscular [kəˈpʌskjulə] *a.* 微粒子的，小体的；血球的

atypical [eɪˈtɪpɪkəl] *a.* not typical or usual 非典型的，不同寻常的

malabsorption [ˌmæləbˈsɔːpʃən] *n.* a failure of absorption, esp. by the small intestine in coeliac disease, cystic fibrosis, etc (由腹部疾病中的小肠、囊性纤维变性等引发的) 吸收障碍

chromosomal [ˌkrəʊməˈsəʊməl] *a.* of or relating to a chromosome 染色体的

jejunal [dʒiˈdʒunə] *a.* 空肠的

biopsy [ˈbaɪɒpsi] *n.* 活组织检查，活体检视

intra-epithelial [ˈɪntrəˌepiˈθiːliəl] *a.* 上皮内的

marrow [ˈmærəʊ] *n.* the soft fatty substance in the hollow centre of bones 骨髓

leukocyte [ˈljuːkəusaɪt] *n.* blood cells that engulf and digest bacteria and fungi; an important part of the body's defense system 白细胞

aeruginosa [ˈɪəruːdʒɪnəʊzə] *n.* 假单胞菌

trephine [trɪˈfaɪn] *a.* a surgical instrument used to remove sections of bone from the skull 环锯，环锯术

hypocellular [haɪpəʊˈseljʊlə] *a.* 细胞减少的

megakaryocytes [mɛgækæriəˈsɪts] *n.* [生物学] 巨核细胞

modality [məʊˈdæləti] *n.* a classification of propositions on the basis of whether they claim necessity or possibility or impossibility 形式，形态

platelet [ˈpleɪtlɪt] *n.* tiny bits of protoplasm found in vertebrate blood; essential for blood clotting [组织] 血小板；薄片

Exercise

Decide whether the following statements are true (T) or false(F) according to the passage.

_____1. The patient had had six episodes of loose stools per day for 3 months accompanied by loss of appetite.

_____2. The girl's liver function, renal function, and urine were tested and their results were normal.

_____3. The girl presented in October 2016 with productive cough, fever, respiratory distress for 3 months, and a history of recurrent infections over the past year.

_____4. The patient was put on a gluten-free diet and supplemented with multivitamins, vitamin C, and iron during her treatment.

_____5. The patient's parents had to deny the doctors' advice to treat with a bone marrow transplantation because of their financial reason.

Answer the following questions according to the passage.

1. What are the girl's symptoms when she presented in Oct. 2013?
_____

2. Should CD always be considered in patients with hematological abnormalities even without any gastrointestinal manifestations (atypical CD)? Why?
_____

3. In your opinions, what treatment is likely to improve the patient's prognosis?
_____

Use the appropriate form of the words or phrases in the box to complete the following sentences.

jejuna	platelet	trephine	atypical	biopsy
asthmatic	marrow	pallor	malabsorption	
modality	adopt	intraepithelial	corpuscular	

1. _____ can be caused by infection, surgery, certain drugs, heavy alcohol use, and digestive disorders such as celiac sprue and Crohn's disease.

2. Where do we draw the line between normal, healthy, typical behavior and what we might want to call abnormal, _____ deviant, unhealthy maladaptive mental problems?

3. Symptoms of anemia include tiredness, lack of stamina, breathlessness, headaches,

insomnia, loss of appetite and _____.

4. Any new prevention _____ must not undermine existing protective behaviors and prevention strategies that reduce the risk of HIV transmission.

5. Von Willebrand disease is characterized primarily by a defect in _____ adhesion to the endothelium.

6. The idea is to pinpoint athletes who might experience _____ symptoms or other breathing problems because of poor air quality.

7. Dysplasia of prostate or prostatic _____ neoplasia (PIN) is associated with prostatic adenocarcinoma, which is quite common in elderly males.

8. Thalassemia can be cured by a successful bone- _____ transplant, however this procedure is expensive and not readily available in most settings.

9. But in a recent Canadian television interview, when the questioner pushed Maggie on whether they euthanized _____ animals, she acknowledged: "If we get them and cannot find them a home, absolutely."

10. The system can be used to count red-cells, white-cells and blood platelets as well as hematocrits and mean _____ volume.

Translation

A. Translate the following expressions into English.

1. 输血   2. 骨髓活组织检查
3. 凝血病组合检查   4. 染色体断裂发生率
5. 空肠切片   6. 高分辨率 CT
7. 无显著特点的瘀斑   8. 抗核抗体

B. Translate the following sentences or expressions into Chinese.

1. The patient had had six or seven episodes of loose stools per day for 3 months accompanied by loss of appetite.

2. There was pallor, multiple generalized petechiae, and eczematous patches on upper back and behind her ears with typical Fanconi facies including microcephaly and microphthalmia.

3. The patient was managed with antibiotics, packed red cells, and platelet support and was put on a gluten-free diet.

4. A bone marrow trephine biopsy was done after consent that revealed hypocellular bone marrow with decreased lymphoid cells, plasma cells, erythroid and myeloid precursors with occasional megakaryocytes.

5. The patient is managed with packed red cells, platelet support, and a gluten-free diet; she showed an increasing trend in platelet count on last follow up.

Section C   Vocabulary (Terminology)

1. 血 blood

Combining form	Meaning	Terminology	Terminology meaning
hem/o	blood	hemolysis	lysis of red blood cells with liberation of hemoglobin 溶血现象，血细胞溶解
heamt/o	blood	hematocrit	the ratio of the volume of red blood cells to the total volume of blood as determined by separation of red blood cells from the plasma usually by centrifugation 血细胞比容

2. 血红蛋白 hemoglobin

Combining form	Meaning	Terminology	Terminology meaning
hemoglobin/o	hemoglobin	hemoglobinopathy	a blood disorder (as sickle-cell anemia) caused by a genetically determined change in the molecular structure of hemoglobin 血红蛋白病

3. 细胞 cell

Combining form	Meaning	Terminology	Terminology meaning
cyt/o	cell	cytokine	any of a class of immunoregulatory proteins (as interleukin or interferon) that are secreted by cells especially of the immune system 细胞因子

4. 红色的 red

Combining form	Meaning	Terminology	Terminology meaning
erythr/o	red	erythrocyte	a cell that contains hemoglobin and can carry oxygen to the body, also called a red blood cell (RBC) 红细胞

5. 红的，玫瑰红的 red, rosy

Combining form	Meaning	Terminology	Terminology meaning
eosin/o	red, rosy	eosinophil	granulocyte readily stained by eosin that is present at sites of allergic reactions and parasitic infections 嗜酸性细胞，嗜伊红细胞

6. 颜色 color

Combining form	Meaning	Terminology	Terminology meaning
chrom/o	color	hypochromic	marked by or being red blood cells with deficient hemoglobin 血蛋白过少的，着色不足的

7. 碱性的，含碱的 base, alkaline

Combining form	Meaning	Terminology	Terminology meaning
bas/o	base, alkaline	basophil	a basophilic substance or structure; *especially*: a white blood cell containing basophilic granules that is similar in function to a mast cell 嗜碱性粒细胞

8. （血等的）凝块 clotting

Combining form	Meaning	Terminology	Terminology meaning
coagul/o	clotting	anticoagulant	a substance that hinders the clotting of blood, blood hinder 抗凝血剂
thromb/o	clot	thromboplastin	a complex enzyme found especially in platelets that functions in the conversion of prothrombin into thrombin in the clotting of blood 凝血激酶

9. 细胞核 nucleus

Combining form	Meaning	Terminology	Terminology meaning
kary/o	nucleus	megakaryocyte	a large cell that has a lobulated nucleus, is found especially in the bone marrow, and is the source of blood platelets 巨核细胞
nucle/o	nucleus	mononuclear	having only one nucleus 单核的

10. 相同，相等 same, equal

Combining form	Meaning	Terminology	Terminology meaning
is/o	same, equal	anisocytosis	an abnormality of red blood cells:they are of unequal size 红细胞大小不均 -cytosis means an increase in the number of cells.

11. 白色的 white

Combining form	Meaning	Terminology	Terminology meaning
Leuk/o	white	leukocyte	White blood cell 白细胞

12. 形态 shape, form

Combining form	Meaning	Terminology	Terminology meaning
morph/o	Shape, form	morphology	a branch of biology that deals with the form and structure of animals and plants or the form and structure of an organism or any of its parts 形态学

13. 中性的 neutral

Combining form	Meaning	Terminology	Terminology meaning
neutr/o	neutral	neutropenia	leukopenia in which the decrease in white blood cells is chiefly in neutrophils 嗜中性白细胞减少症

14. 一、单个的 one, single

Combining form	Meaning	Terminology	Terminology meaning
mon/o	one, single	monocyte	a large white blood cell with finely granulated chromatin dispersed throughout the nucleus that is formed in the bone marrow, enters the blood, and migrates into the connective tissue where it differentiates into a macrophage 巨噬细胞

15. 吃、吞下、咽下 eat, swallow

Combining form	Meaning	Terminology	Terminology meaning
phag/o	eat, swallow	phagocyte	a cell (as a white blood cell) that engulfs and consumes foreign material (as microorganisms) and debris 吞噬细胞

16. 变化，异常 varied, irregular

Combining form	Meaning	Terminology	Terminology meaning
poikil/o	varied, irregular	poikilocyte	异形（红）血球

17. 铁 iron

Combining form	Meaning	Terminology	Terminology meaning
sider/o	iron	siderosis	铁质沉着

18. 球，圆 globe, round

Combining form	Meaning	Terminology	Terminology meaning
shper/o	globe, round	spherocyte	球形细胞

19. 除去，移走 removal，carry away

Combining form	Meaning	Terminology	Terminology meaning
-apheresis	removal, carry away	plasmapheresis	a procedure designed to deplete the body of blood plasma (the liquid part of the blood) without depleting the body of its blood cells 血浆除去法

20.–blast (immature, embryonic)

Combining form	Meaning	Terminology	Terminology meaning
-blast	immature, embryonic	erythroblast	a polychromatic nucleated cell of red bone marrow that synthesizes hemoglobin and that is an intermediate in the initial stage of red blood cell formation; broadly: a cell ancestral to red blood cells 成红细胞

21. -cytosis (abnormal condition of cells, increase in cells)

Combining form	Meaning	Terminology	Terminology meaning
-cytosis	abnormal condition of cells, increase in cells	macrocytosis	the occurrence of macrocytes in the blood 大红细胞症

22. -emia, blood condition

Combining form	Meaning	Terminology	Terminology meaning
-emia	blood condition	leukemia	an acute or chronic disease in humans and other warm-blooded animals characterized by an abnormal increase in the number of white blood cells in the tissues and often in the blood 白血病

23. 蛋白 protein

Combining form	Meaning	Terminology	Terminology meaning
-globin	protein	hemoglobin	an iron-containing respiratory pigment of vertebrate red blood cells that consists of a globin composed of four subunits each of which is linked to a heme molecule, that functions in oxygen transport to the tissues after conversion to oxygenated form in the gills or lungs, and that assists in carbon dioxide transport back to the gills or lungs after surrender of its oxygen 血红蛋白
-globulin		immunoglobulin	

24. 破坏、毁灭的 pertaining to destruction

Combining form	Meaning	Terminology	Terminology meaning
-lytic	pertaining to destruction	thrombolytic	Used to dissolve clots 血栓溶解的，血栓溶解剂

25. 病态、异常状态 osis (abnormal condition)

Combining form	Meaning	Terminology	Terminology meaning
-osis	abnormal condition	thrombosis	the formation of a clot or thrombus within the lumen of a blood vessel, obstructing the flow of blood through the circulatory system 血栓形成

26. 所示物质数目的异常减少 -penia (deficiency)

Combining form	Meaning	Terminology	Terminology meaning
-penia	deficiency	granulocytopenia	A marked decrease in the number of granulocytes 粒细胞缺乏症

27. 吃或食 -phage (eat, swallow)

Combining form	Meaning	Terminology	Terminology meaning
-phage	eat, swallow	macrophage	A type of white blood cell that ingests (takes in) foreign material 巨噬细胞

28. 爱、亲、吸引 -philia（attraction for (an increase in cell numbers)）

Combining form	Meaning	Terminology	Terminology meaning
-philia	attraction for (an increase in cell number)	eosinophilia	an abnormally high number of eosinophils in the blood 嗜酸细胞增多

29. 携运、电泳现象 -phoresis(carrying, transmission)

Combining form	Meaning	Terminology	Terminology meaning
-phoresis	carry	electrophoresis	a process by which molecules (such as proteins, DNA, or RNA fragments) can be separated according to size and electrical charge by applying an electric current to them. Each kind of molecule travels through the medium at a different rate, depending on its electrical charge and molecular size 电泳

30. 产生，形成 -poiesis (formation)

Combining form	Meaning	Terminology	Terminology meaning
-poiesis	formation	hematopoiesis	the production of all types of blood cells generated by a remarkable self-regulated system that is responsive to the demands put upon it 造血

31. 静态 -stasis (stop, control)

Combining form	Meaning	Terminology	Terminology meaning
-stasis	stop, control	hemostasis	the stoppage of bleeding or hemorrhage. Also, the stoppage of blood flow through a blood vessel or organ of the body 止血

Exercise for vocabulary

Match the following pathological conditions or terms with their meanings below.

phagocyte	hematopoiesis	electrophoresis	granulocytopenia
hemolysis	cytokine	erythrocyte	hemoglobinopathy
thrombosis	hematocrit	macrophage	eosinophilia
thromboplastin	neutropenia	thrombolytic	basophil
hemoglobin	leukocyte	macrocytosis	megakaryocyte

_____1. A large cell that has a lobulated nucleus, is found especially in the bone marrow, and is the source of blood platelets.

_____2. Lysis of red blood cells with liberation of hemoglobin.

_____3. A cell (as a white blood cell) that engulfs and consumes foreign material (as microorganisms) and debris.

_____4. A process by which molecules (such as proteins, DNA, or RNA fragments) can be separated according to size and electrical charge by applying an electric current to them. Each kind of molecule travels through the medium at a different rate, depending on its electrical charge and molecular size.

_____5. A marked decrease in the number of granulocytes.

_____6. Any of a class of immunoregulatory proteins (as interleukin or interferon) that are secreted by cells especially of the immune system.

_____7. A blood disorder (as sickle-cell anemia) caused by a genetically determined change in the molecular structure of hemoglobin.

_____8. A cell that contains hemoglobin and can carry oxygen to the body. Also called a red blood cell (RBC).

_____9. The formation of a clot or thrombus within the lumen of a blood vessel, obstructing the flow of blood through the circulatory system.

_____10. Leukopenia in which the decrease in white blood cells is chiefly in neutrophils.

_____11. The occurrence of macrocytes in the blood.

_____12. An iron-containing respiratory pigment of vertebrate red blood cells that consists of a globin composed of four subunits each of which is linked to a heme molecule, that functions in oxygen transport to the tissues after conversion to oxygenated form in the gills or lungs, and that assists in carbon dioxide transport back to the gills or lungs after surrender of its oxygen.

_____13. An abnormally high number of eosinophils in the blood.

_____14. The ratio of the volume of red blood cells to the total volume of blood as determined by separation of red blood cells from the plasma usually by centrifugation.

_____15. The production of all types of blood cells generated by a remarkable self-regulated system that is responsive to the demands put upon it.

_____16. A type of white blood cell that ingests (takes in) foreign material.

_____17. Used to dissolve clots.

_____18. A complex enzyme found especially in platelets that functions in the conversion of prothrombin into thrombin in the clotting of blood.

_____19. A basophilic substance or structure; especially: a white blood cell containing basophilic granules that is similar in function to a mast cell.

_____20. White blood cell.

Choose the term that best completes the meaning of the sentence.

1. A 22-year-old unmarried female presented with dizziness and fatigue for half

a year, the duration of menstrual period lasts 7~8 days with blood clot, the outpatient laboratory findings show: RBC count 3.0×10^{12}/L, hemoglobulin 65g/L, serum ferritin 10μg/L, serum folic acid, VitB$_{12}$ 600pg/L, reticulocyte:0.015. What's the most likely diagnosis?

    A. Megaloblastic anemia.   B. Hemolytic anemia.

    C. Iron deficiency anemia.   D. Aplastic anemia.

2. A 20-year-old student presents your office complaining of a fever and throat. Routine blood test shows a WBC of 28,000 per mm^3 with 95% myeloblasts (polys are 5%). Platelet count is 15000 per mm^3, hemoglobin is 10g/dL. Hematocrit is 22.5. What is your diagnosis?

    A. Autoimmune hemolytic anemia.   B. Thalassemia.

    C. Acute myelogenous leukemia.   D. Chronic lymphocytic leukemia.

3. A married male, aged 36, with history of acute icteric hepatitis was admitted to hospital on June 18th, 2006 complaining of fever and bleeding gum for half a month. On physical examination: severe pallor complexion, the liver palpable 2 cm below the coastal margin and the spleen palpable just below the coastal margin. Laboratory findings show: RBC $\times 10^{12}$/L, hemoglobin 55 g/L. WBC count 2.5×10^9/L, platelet 32×10^9/L, hematocrit 0.002. What's the most likely diagnosis?

    A. Anemia due to chronic hepatopathy (liver diseases).

    B. Megaloblastic anemia.

    C. Aplastic anemia.

    D. Hypersplenism.

4. A 49-year-old male complained of cold intolerance and fever for 13 days. On physical examination: sag in spirit, T 39.5℃, BP 80/50mmHg, purpura found in the right upper limb, respiration 30/min, noisy breathing sound heard on both bottoms of lung, the liver not palpable beneath the coastal margin, the spleen just palpable below the left coastal margin. Laboratory findings shows: Hb 112g/L, WBC 18×10^9/L. platelet 56×10^9/L, PT 17s, fibrinogen 1390 mg/L. What's the most likely diagnosis is?

    A. Acute leukemia.

    B. Pneumonia.

    C. DIC (disseminated intravascular coagulation).

    D. Infection with DIC.

5. A 14-year-old female presented with low-grade fever and arthralgia over the body for 1 week, on physical examination: enlarged lymph node palpable on both sides of neck. The liver and spleen palpable 2 cm below the coastal margin, laboratory findings show: N 30%, L 70%, platelet 20×10^9/L, what's the most likely diagnosis?

    A. Rheumatic fever.   B. SLE.

C. Acute leukemia.　　　　　　　　　D. Malignant lymphoma.

6. While taking coumadin, a blood thinner, Mr. Ratzan's physician made sure to check his _____.

　A. prothrombin time　　　　　　　B. hematocrit

　C. sed rate　　　　　　　　　　　　D. blood sugar

7. When they checked Babette's blood type during her prenatal examination, she was AB-. Her physician told her that she and her baby might have the condition of _____.

　A. Rh incompatibility　　　　　　　B. multiple myeloma

　C. pernicious anemia　　　　　　　D. hypothyroidism

8. While in the hospital, Mr. Klein was told he had an elevated _____ count with a "left shift." This was information that confirmed his diagnosis of systemic infection.

　A. red blood cell　　　　　　　　　B. white blood cell

　C. platelet　　　　　　　　　　　　D. eosinophil

9. Bill as a 10-year-old boy who suddenly noticed many black and blue marks all over his legs. He had a fever and was tired all the time. The physician did a blood test that revealed pancytopenia. A bone marrow biopsy confirmed the diagnosis of _____.

　A. acute lymphocytic leukemia　　　B. polycythemia vera

　C. aplastic anemia　　　　　　　　　D. thyroiditis

10. Dr. Harris experiencing highly heavy menstrual periods. Because of the bleeding, she frequently felt tire and weak and was probably sideropenic. Her physician performed blood tests that revealed her problem as_____.

　A. thrombocytopenia　　　　　　　B. pernicious anemia

　C. iron-deficiency anemia　　　　　D. primary aldosteronism

Section D　Writing

Finding of Laboratory

实验室检查 / 数据资料

实验室检查包括：

1. 可得到的血液检查，如：全血细胞计数、化学检查、肝功能、凝血功能等；

2. 尿液分析；

3. 胸片检查（其他影像学检查）；

4. 心电图；

5. 其他可得到的资料。

Example 1

UA：Clear yellow, PH6.0, specific gravity:1.005. Trace protein1+blood. Neg. nitrites/leukocyte esterase. 2-5 rbc/hpf (high power field).

X-ray: No infiltrates, borderline cardiomegaly, no acute disease.

ECG: NSR (normal sinus rhythm), with normal axis and intervals. No acute ST or T wave abnormalities. No Q waves.

Example 2

Laboratory studies: Results of laboratory investigations revealed the following: white blood cell count, 35.5×10^3 cells/mcl (with 46% neutrophils, 8% lymphocytes, 3% monocytes, 8% eosinophils, and 34% bands); hemoglobin, 8.2 g/dL; mean corpuscular volume, 79.8 FL; red (cell) distribution width (RDW), 15%; platelets, 525×10^3 cells; iron, 12 mcg/dL; transferrin, < 70 mg/dL; ferritin, 565 ng/mL; reticulocyte count, 1.6%; and albumin, 2.4 g/dL.

Example 3

The hemoglobin level was 11.8 g per deciliter and the hematocrit 33.6 percent. Laboratory measurements of the levels of blood chemicals yielded the following results: alanine aminotransferase, 58 U per liter; aspartate aminotransferase, 38 U per liter; and alkaline phosphatase, 118 U per liter. The level of CA-125 was 49.6 U per milliliter. The results of other laboratory tests were within normal ranges.

Exercise

Write the following finding of Laboratory.

患者入院前 2 周，右胁突发剧痛，向腹股沟放射，伴有血尿。5 小时后，患者求诊于家庭附近急诊。体温 36.9℃，血压 142/76mmHg，脉搏 96 次 / 分，呼吸 24 次 / 分，静脉肾盂造影示收集系统扩张，右侧输尿管无对比物质，诊断为右侧肾结石。给予二氢吗啡酮和酮咯酸氨丁三醇止痛，异丙嗪止呕。尿液分析：pH 值 7.5，尿中潜血 +++，红细胞多得无法计算，未见白细胞及细菌。治疗后病情好转，但 7 小时后疼痛再次发作，伴有上腹部不适，寒战，发热，温度达 38.5℃，予以止痛及止呕药，氧氟沙星和法莫替丁后转至医院。

病史小结（病历摘要）

病史小结必须是记录思考鉴别诊断的全过程，列出支持或否定鉴别诊断的资料。在病史小结中有以下几点要注意：

1. 证实你的思维过程；

2. 不要总结，要分析；

3. 以引导的方式涵盖病历中的关键因素，引导阅读病历者进行鉴别诊断，并向阅读病历者引出你的结论；

4. 形成一个疾病列表，并解释说明发生这种状况的原因及发展过程；

5. 用完整的语句叙述。

Example: In summary, the patient is 46 years old, male, with a long history of difficult-control Crohn's diseases who presents with complaints of 3 days of fevers, abdominal bloating and pain and frequent bloody stools after tapering down his mesalamine dose. His exam revealed a mild fever, mild-moderate dehydration (orthostatic hypotension, dry mouth, flat jugular veins, contraction alkalosis and preretinal azotemia), moderate right-sided abdominal tenderness with voluntary guarding, and occult blood-positive stools. His labs show an elevated white blood cell count and mild anemia. Notably, this presentation is similar to his prior Crohn's fares, and it seems most likely that this is recurrence due to recent tapering of his maintenance medicine.

Other possibilities include:

1. Infectious diarrhea (the patient's recent vacation in Mexico puts him at risk for agents like E. Coli and Salmonella).

2. Appendicitis (with a trio of fever, elevated white blood count, and right lower quadrant pain), and incarcerated inguinal hernia. (Small sliding hernia noted on exam-easily reduced).

Less likely concerns wound be:

1. Nephrolithiasis (the pain was not colicky and UA showed no blood. But Crohn's patients are at increased risk for oxalate stones due to augmented GI uptake of oxalate rom abnormal calcium absorption).

2. Pancreatitis (the patient denies a significant ethanol consumption, and gallstone-related diseases is unlikely as he is status post cholecystectomy. Also, blood in stool generally is not seen with pancreatitis).

3. Herpes zoster (It's possible to have zoster without rash, but the distribution of the pain is not strictly dermatomal).

Section E   Spoken English

Role play

Directions: A Child's skin was scattered by a patch of bruise after he got upper respiratory tract infection. 2 students work in pairs to demonstrate the conversation, one plays the role of doctor, the other of child's parent.

Discussion

Directions: Work in groups and discuss with your partners, then answer the following questions with detailed analysis.

A 32-year-old woman is evaluated for fever, chills, and weakness. She had a blood transfusion 10 days prior after she underwent an open reduction and internal fixation of the right femur due to a motor vehicle accident. She has had no significant past medical history except for a C-section 2 years ago at which time she successfully received a blood transfusion.

On examination, she has a fever of 100.1 ℉, blood pressure is 100/64 mmHg, pulse rate is 110 bpm, and respiration is 20/min. On physical examination, the patient appears uncomfortable and has scleral icterus. The remainder of the examination is unremarkable. There is no evidence of bleeding.

Hemoglobin concentration is 6.2 g/dL compared with a hemoglobin of 8.6 g/dL previously. Platelet and leukocyte count are normal. Direct and indirect Coombs tests are positive. The blood bank identifies a new alloantibody on further testing.

1. What is the most likely diagnosis?

2. What is the next step in management?

Terminology in blood department

hemolytic anemia 溶血性贫血

hereditary spherocytosis 遗传性球形细胞增多症

hemoglobinopathy 血红蛋白病

autoimmune hemolytic anemia 自身免疫性溶血性贫血

paroxysmal nocturnal hemoglobinuria 阵发性睡眠性血红蛋白尿

granulocytopenia 粒细胞减少症

agranulocytosis 粒细胞缺乏症

myelodysplastic syndrome 骨髓增生异常综合征

leukemia 白血病

acute leukemia 急性白血病

chronic granulocytic leukemia 慢性粒细胞白血病

chronic lymphocytic leukemia 慢性淋巴细胞白血病

lymphoma 淋巴瘤

plasma cell dyscrasia 浆细胞病

multiple myeloma 多发性骨髓瘤

myeloproliferative disorders 骨髓增生性疾病

primary myelofibrosis 原发性骨髓纤维化症

hypersplenism 脾功能亢进

vascular purpura 血管性紫癜

allergic purpura 过敏性紫癜

hereditary hemorrhagic telangiectasis 遗传性出血性毛细血管扩张症

simple purpura 单纯性紫癜

thrombocytopenia purpura 血小板减少性紫癜

hemophilia 血友病

disseminated intravascular coagulation 弥散性血管内凝血

thrombosis 血栓形成

thromboembolism 血栓栓塞

complete blood cell (CBC) 全血细胞

routine blood test 血常规检查

white blood cell count 白细胞计数

red blood cell count 红细胞计数

reticulocyte count 网织红细胞计数

platelet count 血小板计数

eosinocyte count 嗜酸性粒细胞计数

hemoglobin 血红蛋白

hematocrit 红细胞比容

WBC differential count 白细胞分类

mean corpuscular count 平均红细胞容积

mean corpuscular hemoglobin (MCH) 平均红细胞血红蛋白含量

mean corpuscular hemoglobin concentration (MCHC) 平均红细胞血红蛋白浓度

crenocyte 皱缩红细胞

schistocyte 裂片红细胞

acanthocyte 棘形红细胞

cacryocyte 泪滴状红细胞

spherocyte 球形红细胞

elliptocyte 椭圆形红细胞

sickle cell 镰刀形细胞

target cell 靶形红细胞

toxic granulation 毒性颗粒

neutrophil shift to the left 中性粒细胞核左移

neutrophil shift to the right 中性粒细胞核右移

erythrocyte sedimentation rate (ESR) 血沉

basophilic granulocyte 嗜碱性粒细胞

monocyte 单核细胞

lymphocyte　淋巴细胞

myeloblast　原粒细胞

promyelocyte　早幼粒细胞

myelocyte　中幼粒细胞

metamyelocyte　晚幼粒细胞

band granulocyte　杆状核粒细胞

polymorphonuclears　多形核粒细胞

neutrophil granulocyte　中性粒细胞

basophil granulocyte　嗜碱性粒细胞

eosinophil granulocyte　嗜酸性粒细胞

pronormoblast　原红细胞

basophilic pronormoblast　早幼红细胞

polychromatophilic normoblast　中幼红细胞

orthochromatic normoblast　晚幼红细胞

lymphoblast　原淋巴细胞

prolymphocyte　幼淋巴细胞

lymphocyte　淋巴细胞

monoblast　原单核细胞

promonocyte　幼单核细胞

monocyte　单核细胞

plasmablast　原浆细胞

proplasmacyte　幼浆细胞

plasmacyte　浆细胞

megakaryoblast　原巨核细胞

promegakaryocyte　幼巨核细胞

granular megakaryocyte　颗粒巨核细胞

platelet-producing megakaryocyte　产血小板巨核细胞

iron staining of bone marrow smear　骨髓铁染色

peroxidase staining megakaryocyte　产血小板巨核细胞

iron staining of bone marrow smear　骨髓铁染色

peroxidase staining(POX)　过氧化酶染色

sudan black staining(SB)　苏丹黑染色

alkaline phosphatase staining(ALP)　碱性磷酸酶染色

acid phosphatase staining(ACP)　酸性磷酸酶染色

nonspecific esterase(NSE)　非特异性酯酶

heated normal saline test　热盐水溶解试验

ink phagocytosis test　墨汁吞噬试验

lysozyme staining　溶菌酶染色

serum iron assay　血清铁测定

total iron binding capacity assay　总铁结合力测定

serum ferritin assay　血清铁蛋白测定

serum transferrin assay　血清转铁蛋白测定

vitamin B_{12} assay　维生素 B_{12} 测定

folic acid assay　叶酸测定

osmotic fragility test of erythrocytes　红细胞渗透脆性试验

biochemical assay of pyruvate kinase　丙酮酸激酶的生化测定

methemoglobin reduction test　高铁血红蛋白还原试验

reduced glutathione assay(GSH)　还原型谷胱甘肽测定

glutathione stability test　谷胱甘肽稳定试验

Heinz bodies staining　变性珠蛋白小体染色

heat instability test　热不稳定试验

isopropanol stability test　异丙醇试验

RBC sickling test　红细胞镰变试验

hemoglobin C test　血红蛋白 C 试验

Hb absorption spectrum determination　血红蛋白吸收光谱测定

hemoglobin electrophoresis　血红蛋白电泳

anti-human globulin test (Coombs test)　人球蛋白试验

cold agglutinin assay　冷凝集素测定

cold hemolytic test (Donath-Landsteiner test)　冷溶血试验

heat hemolysis test　热溶血试验

measurement of free Hb levels in plasma　血浆游离血红蛋白测定

urinary hemosiderin determination (Rous test)　尿含铁血黄素检查

platelet count　血小板计数

bleeding time (BT)　出血时间

capillary fragility test　毛细血管脆性试验

examination of capillary in nail fold with microscopy　甲床毛细血管镜检查

assay of malondialdehyde for determination of platelet life-span　丙二醛法测定血小板寿命

platelet adhesion test(PAdT)　血小板粘附试验

platelet aggregation test (PagT)　血小板聚集试验

platelet factor assay　血小板因子测定

β-thromboglobulin (β-TG) assay　β- 血小板球蛋白测定

thromboxane A2(TXA2)assay　血小板血栓烷 A2 测定

clot retraction quantitative assay　血块收缩定量测定

coagulation time (CT) 凝血时间

factor ⅤⅢ coagulant activity 因子ⅤⅢ凝血活性测定

prothrombin time (PT) 凝血酶原时间

recalcification time (RT) 复钙时间

activated coagulation time (ACT) 活化的凝血时间

fibrin peptide A (FPA) 纤维蛋白肽

fibrin plate test 纤维蛋白平板溶解试验

plasma plasminogen assay 血浆纤溶酶原测定

thrombin time (TT) 凝血酶时间

paracoagulation test 副凝试验

staphylococcal clumping test (SCT) 萄葡球菌聚集试验

immunological assay of fibrin-fibrinogen degradation products 纤维蛋白（原）降
解产物的免疫学测定

D-dimer fragments assay D- 二聚体测定

α2-macroglobulin (α2-MG)assay α2- 巨球蛋白测定

antithrombin Ⅲ (AT-Ⅲ) assay 抗凝血酶Ⅲ测定

Chapter 10

Obstetric & Gynecological System

Section A   Focus Listening

Conversation

Listen to the dialogue and fill in the blanks with proper words.

D=doctor P=patient

D: What seems to be the problem?

P: I have been getting terribly crampy feeling in my lower abdomen, nausea, abdominal bloating, _____ and constipation.

D: Do you have history of _____ disease?

P: No, not that I know of.

D: Do you have _____, depression, distending pain in breast?

P: Yes, I do.

D: Do you have a regular cycle?

P: Yes, it's quite regular and comes about every 28 days.

D: How long does your period last?

P: Usually about 5 to 6 days.

D: Is your period quite light, average or heavy?

P: It's about moderate. Doctor.

D: Have you been passing any _____ in them?

P: Well, there were one or two clots in every period last year, but I did not have any this year.

D: Do these discomforts present prior to or after the period?

P: They come on prior to the periods, usually in the middle of period.

D: Any other symptoms?

P: I get uptight, irritability, depression, anxiety and edema of limbs just before my period. I often find I gain weight before it.

D: Do these symptoms disappear as soon as the bleeding begins?

P: Yes, they do.

D: That sounds typical of premenstrual tension.

P: Premenstrual tension?

D: Yes. Premenstrual tension, called premenstrual _____, is a diverse constellation of cyclic physical and emotional symptoms, occurring monthly during the luteal phase of the menstrual cycle. Don't worry. There are some pamphlets on premenstrual tension available if you ask the nurse.

New Words & Expressions

cramp 痛性痉挛   constellation 群集
flatulence 胃肠胀气   luteum 黄体
period 月经   luteal 黄体的
clot 血块   pamphlet 小册子
up-tight 烦躁的，急躁的，不安的

Passage

Answer the questions after listening to the passage.

1. Which of the following is NOT related to PCOS?

A. Delay in menstruation.   B. Heavy bleeding.

C. Excess hair on the body.   D. Respiratory distress.

2. What is the absence of menstruation for more than three months called as?

A. Primary amenorrhea.   B. Oligomenorrhea.

C. Secondary amenorrhea.   D. Oliguria.

3. Which of the following is/are the risky factors of PCOS?

A. Diabetes.   B. Metabolic syndrome.

C. Hypertension.   D. All of the above.

4. Which of the following hormone level is increased in PCOS?

A. Thyroxine.   B. Androgens.

C. Glucagon.   D. Growth hormone.

5. Which of the following best describes the term anovulatory cycles?

A. Menstruation with ovulation.

B. Menstruation without ovulation.

C. Menstruation with ovulation and bleeding.

D. Menstruation without ovulation and heavy bleeding.

Section B   Reading Comprehension

Text

A 34-year-old woman presents to the emergency department (ED) a 2-hour history of severe abdominal pain, 2 episodes of lightheadedness, and loss of consciousness. She states that she is about 6-week pregnancy and that the pain started suddenly in the morning of presentation. She went to the bathroom and sat on the toilet when she felt light-headed. After her second time passing out, she alerted her husband to call for an ambulance. She denies any vaginal bleeding or discharge. There is no nausea or vomiting, and the patient has not experienced any fevers. The patient has visited an obstetrician for prenatal care but has not yet had an ultrasonogram. The patient is currently G3P1011; she had a spontaneous abortion that complicated a prior pregnancy 4 years ago. There is no history of pelvic inflammatory disease or prior ectopic pregnancy. She is currently not undergoing ovulatory induction. She does not have an IUD. The patient has no chronic medical problems and takes no medications regularly. She does not drink alcohol and does not use any illicit substances.

On physical examination, her blood pressure is 86/55 mmHg, and she is noted to be tachycardic, with a regular rhythm at approximately 130 bpm. She has a normal oral temperature of 98.9℉ (37.2℃) and a respiratory rate of 12 breaths/min. She appears pale and visibly frightened. The pulmonary and cardiac examinations are otherwise unremarkable. The patient's abdomen is slightly distended, with diffuse tenderness to palpation that is most severe in the left lower quadrant. An external examination of the perineum is unremarkable for fluid or blood. On pelvic examination, a moderate amount of blood is noted in the vaginal vault, with tenderness to palpation in the left adnexa. The uterus is normal sized. No adnexal masses are palpable. No lower limb edema is noted, and the patient has normal peripheral pulses.

The patient is hooked up to central monitoring and 2 large-bore, peripheral intravenous lines are placed. A complete set of laboratory investigations are sent, and 2 liters of normal saline are rapidly infused. The patient's heart rate responds by decreasing to approximately 99 bpm, and her blood pressure rebounds to 104/55 mmHg. A bedside ultrasonographic examination is performed, and it demonstrates a hypoechoic stripe indicative of free fluid in the right upper quadrant between the liver and the kidney (see

Panel A). As a result, a stat formal ultrasonogram is performed to confirm the finding of the bedside ultrasonogram and to identify a specific etiology for it; in the meantime, a stat obstetric consult is called to prepare the patient for the operating room. Her laboratory tests include a basic metabolic panel; the results are normal. Her complete blood cell (CBC) count shows a low hemoglobin of 7.3 g/dL (73 g/L); a slightly elevated white blood cell (WBC) count of $13.8 \times 10^3/\mu L$ ($13.8 \times 10^9/L$), with a normal differential; and a normal platelet count. The basic metabolic panel is unremarkable. A urine pregnancy test is positive. A coagulation profile and a quantitative β-human chorionic gonadotropin (β-hCG) are drawn. Images of the formal transvaginal ultrasonogram are also presented (see Figure 6).

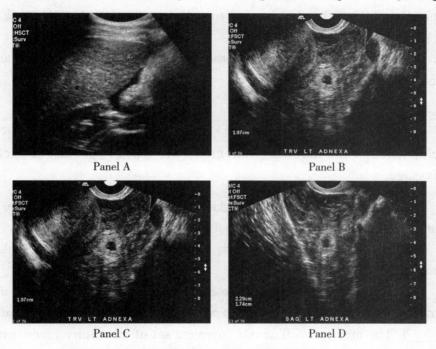

Panel A · Panel B · Panel C · Panel D

Figure 6　Image of formal transvaginal ultrasonogram

New Words & Expressions

light-headedness　*n.* a reeling sensation; a feeling that you are about to fall 头晕眼花
ultrasonogram [ʌltrəˈsɒnəgræm]　*n.* 超声波谱图，超声记录图
ectopic [ekˈtɒpɪk]　*a.* [病理学] 异位的，异常的
ovulatory [ˈəuvjulətəri]　*a.* 排卵的，产卵的
tachycardic [tæki'ka:dik]　*a.* 心搏过速的，心动过速的
distend [dɪˈstend]　*v.* cause to expand as it by internal pressure 使……膨胀；使……扩张
diffuse [dɪˈfju:z]　*a.* spread out; not concentrated in one place 弥漫的；散开的
perineum [ˌperɪˈni:əm]　*n.* the region of the body between the anus and the genital organs, including some of the underlying structures 会阴

adnexa [æd'neksə] *n*. an accessory or adjoining anatomical parts or appendages (especially of the embryo) [解剖] 附件；[动][解剖] 附器（等于 annexa）

peripheral [pə'rɪfərəl] *a*. on or near an edge or constituting an outer boundary; the outer area 外围的；次要的

hypoechoic [haɪ'pəʊkɔɪk] *n*. 低回声

quadrant ['kwɒdrənt] *n*. a quarter of the circumference of a circle 四分之一圆

obstetric [əb'stetrɪk] *a*. of or relating to childbirth or obstetrics 产科的

coagulation[kəu,ægju'leɪʃən] *n*. the process of forming semi solid lumps in a liquid 凝固，凝结物

rupture ['rʌptʃə] *v*. to break or burst, or to make something break or burst（使）破裂，（使）爆裂

placenta [plə'sentə] *n*. an organ that forms inside a woman's uterus to feed an unborn baby [胚] 胎盘

Exercise

Decide whether the following statements are true (T) or false (F) according to the passage.

_____1. The patient, 29-years-old, states that she has been pregnant for about 6 weeks? and that the pain started suddenly in the early morning of presentation.

_____2. The patient doesn't have any chronic medical problems and takes some medications regularly.

_____3. During the patient's pelvic examination, these symptoms, a moderate amount of blood noted in the vaginal vault and pain to palpation in the left adnexa, are found.

_____4. The medical staff sent a complete set of laboratory investigation and quickly instilled 2 liters of normal saline.

_____5. Including a basic metabolic panel, the results of her laboratory tests are abnormal.

Answer the following questions according to the passage.

1. What symptoms did the patient have when she presents to the emergency department?

_____

2. What possibilities can you diagnose from the patient's statement at the beginning?

_____

3. What do the ultrasonographic images demonstrate?

_____

Use the appropriate form of the words or phrases in the box to complete the following sentences.

Ectopic	distend	lightheadedness	coagulation	rupture
peripheral	ultrasonogram	diffuse	pelvicplacenta	
obstetric	spontaneous	identify	distend	

1. Parts of the blood do not work together well creating unneeded _____ related to heart disease or clots.

2. That'll not only give you some _____ practice in talking the stuff but also earn you some "brownie points " for trying really hard.

3. The primary role of AM is to_____ blood vessel and decrease blood pressure, and it can also restrain the migration of vessel smooth muscle cells.

4. The accusation led to a _____ of the company's relationship with China and a decision by Google not to cooperate with China's censorship.

5. In general terms, an _____ pregnancy is a pregnancy that occurs and develops outside of the woman's uterus.

6. The essential thing for _____ countries would be to regain competitiveness and to hopefully run trade surpluses which help their economic growth.

7. In this case, you try to _____ his specific features implemented in the code and then map them to the use cases.

8. They left me dizzy and _____ but I still had enough wits about me to select one brand that tasted good and actually went down easy.

9. The gas became so _____, it could not form nearby stars and solar systems, nor fall back inward to feed black holes.

10. As a result, more trained staffs have been recruited in district health centers in recent years and more pregnant women have gained access to essential _____ care.

Translation

A. Translate the following expressions into English.

1. 胎盘前置   2. 阴道超声波
3. 自然流产   4. 尿妊娠检查
5. 盆腔炎   6. 会阴的外部检查
7. 正常的血小板数   8. 黄体囊肿破裂

B. Translate the following sentences or expressions into Chinese.

1. A bedside ultrasonographic examination is performed, and it demonstrates a hypoechoic stripe indicative of free fluid in the right upper quadrant between the liver and

the kidney.

2. She states that she is about 6 weeks pregnant and that the pain started suddenly in the morning of presentation.

3. The patient's abdomen is slightly distended, with diffuse tenderness to palpation that is most severe in the left lower quadrant.

4. The patient has visited an obstetrician for prenatal care but has not yet had an ultrasonogram.

5. As a result, a stat formal ultrasonogram is performed to confirm the finding of the bedside ultrasonogram and to identify a specific etiology for it.

Section C   Vocabulary (Terminology)

1. 女性 woman, female

Combining form	Meaning	Terminology	Terminology meaning
gynec/o	woman, female	gynecomastia	enlargement of one or both breasts in a male. It often occurs with puberty, aging, or can be drug related 男性乳房发育症
		gynecology	a branch of medicine that deals with the diseases and routine physical care of the reproductive system of women 妇科学
estr/o	female	estrogen	a female hormone produced by the ovaries 雌（甾）激素

2. 助产士 midwife

Combining form	Meaning	Terminology	Terminology meaning
obstetr/o	midwife	obstetrician	a physician specializing in obstetrics 产科医师

3. 怀孕 pregancy

Combining form	Meaning	Terminology	Terminology meaning
-gravida	pregnancy	primigravida	a woman during her first pregnant 初孕
-cyesis	pregnancy	pseudocyesis	a psychosomatic state that occurs without conception and is marked by some of the physical symptoms and changes in hormonal balance of pregnancy 假性怀孕

4. 分娩 childbirth, delivery, labor

Combining form	Meaning	Terminology	Terminology meaning
toc/o	childbirth	oxytocin	a pituitary octapeptide hormone $C_{43}H_{66}N_{12}O_{12}S_2$ that stimulates especially the contraction of uterine muscle and the secretion of milk 催产素

续表

Combining form	Meaning	Terminology	Terminology meaning
nat/i	birth	neonatal	of, relating to, or affecting the newborn and especially the human infant during the first month after birth 新生儿的；初生的
-tocia	labour, birth	oxytocia	Slow and difficult labor or delivery 难产

5. 乳房 breast

Combining form	Meaning	Terminology	Terminology meaning
mamm/o	breast	mammoplasty	乳房成形术
mast/o	breast	mastitis	inflammation of the breast or udder usually caused by infection 乳腺炎

6. 乳，奶 milk

Combining form	Meaning	Terminology	Terminology meaning
lact/o	milk	prolactin	a protein hormone of the anterior lobe of the pituitary that induces lactation 催乳素
galact/o	milk	galactorrhea	a spontaneous flow of milk from the nipple 乳溢

7. 月经 menses, menstruation

Combining form	Meaning	Terminology	Terminology meaning
men/o	menses	amenorrhea	absence or cessation of menstruation 闭经

8. 外阴 vulva

Combining form	Meaning	Terminology	Terminology meaning
episi/o	vulva	episiotomy	surgical incision of the perineum to enlarge the vaginal opening for obstetrical purposes during the birth process 外阴切开术
vulv/o	vulva	vulvovaginitis	coincident inflammation of the vulva and vagina 外阴阴道炎

9. 阴道 vagina

Combining form	Meaning	Terminology	Terminology meaning
colp/o	vigina	colposcopy	a magnifying instrument designed to facilitate visual inspection of the vagina and cervix 阴道镜检查
vagin/o	vagina	vaginitis	inflammation of the vagina 阴道炎

10. 子宫 womb, uterus

Combining form	Meaning	Terminology	Terminology meaning
hyster/o	womb, uterus	hysteroscopy	visual examination of the cervix and interior of the uterus with an endoscope 宫腔镜

Combining form	Meaning	Terminology	Terminology meaning
metr/o	uterus	metrorrhagia	irregular uterine bleeding especially between menstrual periods 子宫出血
metri/o	uterus	endometriosis	the presence of endometrium in areas other than the lining of the uterus, as on the ovaries, resulting in premenstrual pain 子宫内膜异位症
uter/o	uterus	uterocervical	of or relating with uterus and cervix 子宫颈的

11. 子宫颈 cervix, neck

Combining form	Meaning	Terminology	Terminology meaning
cervic/o	cervix, neck	endocervicitis	子宫颈内膜炎

12. 羊膜 amnion

Combining form	Meaning	Terminology	Terminology meaning
amni/o	amnion	amniocentesis	羊膜穿刺术

13. 绒毛膜 chorion

Combining form	Meaning	Terminology	Terminology meaning
chori/o	chorion	choriocarcinoma	a malignant tumor typically developing in the uterus from the trophoblast 绒毛膜癌
chorion/o	chorion	chorionic	of, relating to, or being part of the chorion 绒毛膜的

14. 输卵管 fallopian tube

Combining form	Meaning	Terminology	Terminology meaning
salping/o	fallopian tubes	salpingectomy	surgical removal of fallopian 输卵管切除术
-salpinx	uterine tube	pyosalpinx	输卵管积脓

15. 生（小孩），开（花），结（果）to bear, bring forth

Combining form	Meaning	Terminology	Terminology meaning
-parous	to bear, bring forth	primiparous	an individual bearing a first offspring 初产的；初次分娩的

16. 排出（液体、气体等）discharge

Combining form	Meaning	Terminology	Terminology meaning
-rrhea	discharge	leukorrhea	a whitish viscid discharge from the vagina resulting from inflammation or congestion of the mucous membrane 白带

17. 转位 acting of turning

Combining form	Meaning	Terminology	Terminology meaning
-version	acting of turning	cephalic version	The fetal head turns or is turned toward the cervix 头转位

18. 疼痛的 painful

Combining form	Meaning	Terminology	Terminology meaning
dys-	painful	dyspareunia	painful sexual intercourse 交媾困难

19. 内的，里面的 within, in

Combining form	Meaning	Terminology	Terminology meaning
endo-	within	endometritis	inflammation of the endometrium 子宫内膜炎
intra-	within	intravenous	situated, performed, or occurring within or entering by way of a vein; *also*: used in or using intravenous procedures 静脉内的
in-	in	involution	the regressive alterations of a body or its parts characteristic of the aging process（器官的）退化；衰退

20. 多 many

Combining form	Meaning	Terminology	Terminology meaning
multi-	many	multipara	经产妇

21. 不 no, not, none

Combining form	Meaning	Terminology	Terminology meaning
nulli	not, no, none	nullipara	未产妇

22. 开始 beginning

Combining form	Meaning	Terminology	Terminology meaning
-arche	beginning	menarche	the beginning of the menstrual function; *especially*: the first menstrual period of an individual 月经初潮

23. 在……之前的 before

Combining form	Meaning	Terminology	Terminology meaning
pre-	before	prenatal	occurring, existing, or performed before birth 产前的，出生前的

24. 往后的 backward

Combining form	Meaning	Terminology	Terminology meaning
retro-	backward	retroversion	the uterus is abnormally turned backward 子宫后屈

25. 第一的，首次的 first

Combining form	Meaning	Terminology	Terminology meaning
primi-	first	primipara	an individual bearing a first offspring, or an individual that has borne only one offspring 初次怀孕的妇女

Exercise for vocabulary

Match the following pathological conditions or terms with their meanings below.

gynecology	retroversion	menarche	estrogen	obstetrician
leukorrhea	primigravida	salpingectomy	oxytocin	oxytocia
mastitis	prolactin	lactose	galactorrhea	dysmenorrhea
amenorrhea	vulvovaginitis	colposcopy	hysteroscopy	choriocarcinoma

_____1. A branch of medicine that deals with the diseases and routine physical care of the reproductive system of women.

_____2. Surgical removal of fallopian.

_____3. A spontaneous flow of milk from the nipple.

_____4. A woman during her first pregnant.

_____5. A female hormone produced by the ovaries.

_____6. A protein hormone of the anterior lobe of the pituitary that induces lactation.

_____7. Inflammation of the breast or udder usually caused by infection.

_____8. The uterus is abnormally turned backward.

_____9. A physician specializing in obstetrics.

_____10. Slow and difficult labor or delivery.

_____11. Absence or cessation of menstruation.

_____12. A disaccharide sugar $C_{12}H_{22}O_{11}$ that is present in milk and yields glucose and galactose upon hydrolysis and yields especially lactic acid upon fermentation.

_____13. Painful menstruation.

_____14. A magnifying instrument designed to facilitate visual inspection of the vagina and cervix.

_____15. A malignant tumor typically developing in the uterus from the trophoblast.

_____16. Coincident inflammation of the vulva and vagina.

_____17. A pituitary octapeptide hormone $C_{43}H_{66}N_{12}O_{12}S_2$ that stimulates especially the contraction of uterine muscle and the secretion of milk.

_____18. The beginning of the menstrual function; especially: the first menstrual period of an individual.

_____19. Visual examination of the cervix and interior of the uterus with an endoscope.

_____20. A whitish viscid discharge from the vagina resulting from inflammation or congestion of the mucous membrane.

Choose the term that best completes the meaning of the sentence.

1. Dr. Hanson felt that it was important to do a _____ once yearly on each of her GYN patients to screen for abnormal cells.

   A. culdocentesis   B. Pap smear

   C. amniocentesis   D. leiomyoma of uterus

2. When Doris missed her period, her doctor checked for the presence of _____ in Doris' urine to see if she was pregnant.

   A. LH   B. IUD   C. HCG   D. ATH

3. Ellen was 34 weeks pregnancy, experiencing bad headaches, a 10-pound weight gain in 2 days, and blurry vision. Dr. Murphy told her to go to the obstetrical emergency room because she suspected _____.

   A. preeclampsia   B. pelvic inflammatory disease

   C. fibroids   D. abortion

4. Dr. Harris felt a breast mass when examining Mrs. Clark. She immediately ordered a _____ for her 35-year-old patient.

   A. dilation and curettage   B. hysterosalpingogram

   C. mammogram   D. CT

5. Clara knew that she should not ignore her fevers and yellow vaginal discharge and the pain in her side. She had previous episodes of _____ treated with IV antibiotics. She worried that she might have a recurrent.

   A. PMS   B. PID

   C. DES   D. menopausal (climacteric) syndrome.

6. After years of trying to become pregnant, Jill decided to speak to her _____ about in vitro fertilization.

   A. hematologist   B. gynecologist

   C. urologist   D. surgeon

7. To harvest her ova, Jill's physician prescribed hormones to stimulate egg maturation and ____. Ova were surgically removed and fertilized with sperm cells in a petri dish.

   A. coitus   B. lactation

   C. ovulation   D. starch

8. Multiple embryos were implanted into Jill's _____ and she received hormones to ensure the survival at least one embryo.

   A. fallopian tube   B. vagina

   C. uterus   D. abdomen

9. The IVF was successful and after _____ Jill was told that she would have twins in

8 1/2 months.

    A. abdominal CT   B. ultrasound

    C. pelvimetry   D. mammography

10. At 37 weeks, Jill went into labor. Under continuous _____, two healthy infants were delivered vaginally.

    A. chronic villus sampling   B. culdocentesis

    C. fetal monitoring   D. birth trauma

Section D   Writing

Diagnosis & Treatment Plan

写诊疗计划有三种常用的组织方法：

1. 列出特殊问题。

2. 按顺序列出各个器官系统。

3. 根据相对重要程序列出各个器官系统。

以上三种方法各有优点，第一种方法是先列出问题的标题，然后简述打算解决该问题的方法，很多医生常用这种方法。当你列出标题时，重要的是对于你思考的确切问题要尽可能明确。

我们举例说明：

A 46-year-old male with a long history difficult-to-control Crohn's disease who presents with complaints of 3 days of fever, abdominal bloating and pain, and frequent bloody stools after tapering down his mesalamine dose. His exam revealed a mild fever, mild-moderate dehydration (orthostatic hypotension, dry mouth, flat jugular veins, contraction alkalosis, and prerenal azotemia), moderate right-sided abdominal tenderness with voluntary guarding, and occult, blood-positive stools. His labs show an elevated white blood cell count and mild anemia, notably, this presentation is similar to his prior Crohn's flares, and it seems most likely that this is a recurrence due to recent tapering of his maintenance medicine.

The plan

1. Diffuse abdominal pain:

Obtain CT abdomen looking for abscess or perforation.

Stool for wbc (if +, will culture), and Ova & parasites.

Will discuss with GI restarting patient's prednisone.

Begin IV fluids with potassium supplementation at 250 mL/hr.

Consider oral metronidazole.

Ask surgery to evaluate patient if there is any deterioration.

Control pain with low doses of morphine.

2. Normocytic anemia:

Likely due to anemia of chronic diseases.

At risk for Fe, folate, B_{12} deficiency from Crohn's.

Will check Fe studies, folate, B_{12} and blood smear.

No need for transfusion now.

Monitor Hb/Hct with rehydration –may fall.

Azotemia, likely prerenal.

Likely secondary to volume depletion due to increased stool volume and poor PO intake.

Will follow post hydration.

No evidence of upper GI bleeding to raise BUN.

May need renal ultrasound if not improved with fluids.

3. Heroin use:

At risk for progressing to IV heroin use.

Possible candidate for Hep B vaccination Check Hep B panel.

Will discuss with patient this high-risk behavior.

Social work consults to address drug use.

Diagnostic impression

这部分是医生分析病情所做的诊断。患者刚入院，对病情只能做大致判断。经过住院观察、治疗，才能得出明确判断，即最后诊断。

Example 1

Impression:

Coronary heart disease

Left ventricular hypertrophy

Angina pectoris

印象诊断：

冠心病

左心室肥厚

心绞痛

Example 2

Impression:

Mild diabetes

Urinary tract infection

印象诊断：

中度糖尿病

尿道感染

Exercise

Write the following diagnostic impression.

1. 印象诊断：
风湿性心脏病
二尖瓣狭窄
右心室扩大
心衰
室性期前收缩
2. 印象诊断：
慢性肾盂肾炎急性发作

Section E　Spoken English

Role play

Directions: A patient was suffering from gynecological diseases for a long time and she went to clinic for help. 2 students work in pairs to demonstrate the conversation, one plays the role of doctor, the other of patient.

Discussion

Directions: Work in groups and discuss with your partners, then answer the following questions with detailed analysis.

A 38 years-old woman complains of amenorrhea, and her menarche began at age 12 years and occurred every 28-30 days. However, about 9 months ago, her cycles seemed to be lengthened and for the last 3 months she has not had a period at all. She has milky breast leakage. She had a bilateral tubal ligation after her last pregnancy, and she has no other past medical or surgical history, taking no medications except multivitamins. Over the last year, she thinks she has gained about 10 pounds, suffering fatigue, mild thinning of her hair, and slightly more coarse skin. She denies headaches or visual changes. Her physical exam, including a pelvic exam and breast exam, is normal, and she is not obese or hirsute. You can elicit slight whitish nipple discharge.

1. What is the most likely diagnosis?
2. What is the most likely etiology for the condition?

Terminology in gynecological and obstetric department

vulvitis　外阴炎

chronic vulvar dystrophy　慢性外阴营养不良

pruritus vulvae　外阴瘙痒

leukoderma vulvae　外阴白斑

albinism　白化病

Bartholin's gland cyst (abscess)　前庭大腺囊肿（脓肿）

trichomonas (monilial, senile) vaginitis (colpitis)　滴虫（念珠菌，老年）性阴道炎

cervical erosion (hypertrophy, polyp, cyst)　宫颈糜烂（肥大，息肉，囊肿）

cervicitis　宫颈炎

salpingitis (ovaritis)　输卵管（卵巢）炎

pelvic parametritis　盆腔结缔组织炎

tuberculosis of the ovary (endometrium, pelvic peritoneum, uterine tube)　卵巢（子宫内膜，盆腔腹膜，输卵管）结核

gonorrhea　淋病

papilloma (fibroma, lipoma) of vulva　外阴乳头状瘤（纤维瘤，脂肪瘤）

squamocellular (basal cell) carcinoma of vulva　外阴鳞状上皮（基底）细胞癌

malignant melanoma　恶性黑色素瘤

Paget disease　佩吉特病

Bowen's disease　表皮内癌

cervical carcinoma　宫颈癌

leiomyoma of uterus　子宫平滑肌瘤

submucous (subserous, intramural) myoma　黏膜下（浆膜下，肌壁间）子宫肌瘤

multiple myomata of uterus　多发性子宫肌瘤

leiomyosarcoma　平滑肌肉瘤

carcinoma of endometrium　子宫内膜癌

follicle cyst (teratoma, cystadenoma, corpus luteum) of ovarium　卵巢卵泡囊肿（畸胎瘤，囊腺瘤，黄体囊肿）

carcinoma of the fallopian tube　输卵管癌

heterotopia endometriosis　子宫内膜异位症

polycystic ovary　多囊卵巢

amenorrhea (menopause, dysmenorrhea)　闭（停，痛）经

dysfunctional menstrual disorder　功能失调月经紊乱

premenstrual tension syndrome　经前期紧张综合征

menopausal (climacteric) syndrome　更年期综合征

cystocele (rectocele)　膀胱（直肠）膨出

prolapse of uterus　子宫脱垂

imperforate hymen　处女膜闭锁

congenital absence of vagina (uterus)　先天性无阴道（子宫）

double vagina　双阴道

atresia (stenosis) of vagina　阴道闭锁（狭窄）

transverse (longitudinal) vaginal septum　阴道横（纵）隔

uterine hypoplasia (infantile uterus)　子宫发育不良（幼稚子宫）

double uterus (didelphia)　双子宫

uterus bicornis (unicornis)　双（单）角子宫

primordial (solidary) uterus　始基（实性）子宫

uterus duplex (septum)　重复（纵隔）子宫

ovarian hypoplasia　卵巢发育不良

true (pseudo) hermaphroditism　真（假）两性畸形

infertility　不孕症

ambivalent　两性人

rectovaginal (urethrovaginal, vesicocervical, vesicovaginal, ureterovaginal)　直肠阴道的（尿道阴道的，膀胱宫颈的，膀胱阴道的，输尿管阴道的）

fistula　瘘

hemorrhagic contact　接触性出血

herpes zoster　带状疱疹

(2) 产科疾病 gynecological diseases

threatened (habitual, inevitable) abortion　先兆（习惯，难免）流产

complete (incomplete, missed) abortion　完全（不全，过期）流产

induced (artificial) abortion　人工流产

spontaneous abortion　自然流产

criminal abortion　堕胎

premature birth　早产

extrauterine pregnancy　宫外孕

tubal (abdominal, cervical, ovarian, interstitial) pregnancy　输卵管（腹腔，宫颈，卵巢，间质部）妊娠

hyperemesis gravidarum (morning sickness)　妊娠剧吐（晨吐）

edema-proteinuria hypertension (pregnancy-hypertension) syndrome　妊高征

preeclampsia (eclampsia)　（先兆）子痫

complete (partial, low lying) placenta previa　完全（部分，低置）性前置胎盘

marginal (latae) placenta previa　边缘性前置胎盘

placenta abruption (ablatio placenta)　胎盘早剥

multiple pregnancy　多胎妊娠

monozygotic (dizygotic) twins 单（双）卵双胎

poly-(oligo-) hydramnios 羊水过多（少）

prolonged (delayed) pregnancy 过期妊娠

fetal death (stillbirth) 死胎

stillborn (postmature delivery) 死产

high risk pregnancy 高危妊娠

uterine inertia (over-efficiency) 宫缩乏力（过强）

generally contracted (flat, funnel, deformed) pelvis 均小（扁平，漏斗，畸形）骨盆

transversely (flat) contracted pelvis 横径（扁平）狭窄骨盆

cervical (vulvar) edema 宫颈（外阴）水肿

breech (shoulder, face) presentation 臀（肩，面）先露

transverse lie 横产

fetal macrosomia 巨大胎儿

monster 畸胎

hydrocephalus (anencephalus) 脑积水（无脑儿）

conjoined twins 联体双胎

fetal distress 胎儿窘迫

rupture of uterus 子宫破裂

postpartum hemorrhage due to uterine inertia 产后宫缩乏力性出血

retained (adherent) placenta 胎盘滞留（粘连）

placenta incarcerate (infarction) 胎盘嵌顿（梗塞）

injuries of the soft birth canal 软产道损伤

cervical (colpoperineal) laceration 宫颈（会阴阴道）裂伤

premature rupture of membrane 胎膜早破

prolapse of the umbilical cord 脐带脱垂

umbilical cord round the neck 脐带绕颈

too long (short) umbilical cord 脐带过长（短）

knots (torsion) of umbilical cord 脐带打结（扭转）

amniotic fluid embolism 羊水栓塞

puerperal infection (heatstroke) 产褥感染（中暑）

(malignant) hydatidiform mole （恶性）葡萄胎

choriocarcinoma 绒毛膜癌

antepartum fetal distress 产前胎儿窘迫

asphyxia neonatorum 新生儿窒息

intracranial hemorrhage 颅内出血

cephalohematoma 头颅血肿

painless childbirth 无痛分娩

Rh blood group incompatibility　Rh 血型不合

subinvolution of uterus　子宫复旧不全

induced delivery　引产

galactostasis　乳汁积滞

agalactia　无乳

birth trauma　产伤

aspiration pneumonia　吸入性肺炎

fetus in fetus　胎内胎

difficult (natural) delivery　难（平）产

abdominal (forceps) delivery　剖宫产（产钳分娩）

References

［1］庄启辉，邱陶生 . 高级医学英语［M］. 北京：中国协和医科大学出版社，2001.

［2］董双辰 . 医学专业英语［M］. 北京：人民卫生出版社，2001.

［3］王文秀，唐文彦 . 新世纪医务英语会话［M］. 上海：上海外语教育出版社，2001.

［4］杨明山 . 医学英语快速阅读教程［M］. 上海：上海中医药大学出版社，2002.

［5］王文秀，冯永平 . 英汉对照医务英语会话［M］. 北京：人民卫生出版社，2003.

［6］王文秀，冯永平 . 医务英语应用文集［M］. 北京：人民卫生出版社，2003.

［7］李传英，潘承礼 . 医学英语写作［M］. 武汉：武汉大学出版社，2007.

［8］Steven L.Berk, PreTest Self-assessment and Review［M］. 北京：人民卫生出版社，2001.

［9］Maria Gyorffy. English for doctors［M］. 上海：复旦大学出版社，2005.

［10］Davi Ellen Chabner. 医学英语教程［M］. 北京：北京大学医学部出版社，2006.

［11］Eugene C. Toy, John Patlan, S Elizabeth Cruse.Case files internal medicine［M］. 长沙：湖南科学技术出版社，2006.

［12］Linda.C. Adam.Practical oral medical English［M］. 北京：中国水利水电出版社，2008.

［13］Jeffrey L. Greenwald. Writing a history & physical［M］.Pennsylvania: Elsevier, USA2009.